Water Recreation and Disease

Water Recreation and Disease

Plausibility of Associated Infections: Acute Effects, Sequelae and Mortality

Kathy Pond

Publishing

LONDON • SEATTLE

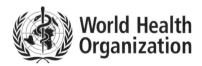
World Health Organization

Published on behalf of the World Health Organization by
IWA Publishing, Alliance House, 12 Caxton Street, London SW1H 0QS, UK

Telephone: +44 (0) 20 7654 5500; Fax: +44 (0) 20 7654 5555; Email: publications@iwap.co.uk
www.iwapublishing.com

First published 2005
© World Health Organization (WHO) 2005

Printed by TJ International (Ltd), Padstow, Cornwall, UK
Index compiled by Indexing Specialists (UK) Ltd, Hove, UK

Disclaimer

British Library Cataloguing-in-Publication Data
A CIP catalogue record for this book is available from the British Library

WHO Library Cataloguing-in-Publication Data
Pond, Kathy.

    Water recreation and disease. Plausibility of Associated Infections: Acute Effects, Sequelae and Mortality / K. Pond
    (Emerging issues in water and infectious diseases series)
    1.Swimming pools 2.Bathing beaches 3.Communicable diseases - transmisssion
    4.Acute disease - epidemiology 5.Water microbiology 6.Disease.reservoirs
    7.Severity of illness index 8.Risk factors I.Title II.Series.
    ISBN 92 4 156305 2   (NLM classification: WA 820)
    ISSN 1728-2160

ISBN 1843390663 (IWA Publishing)

Contents

Foreword

Worldwide, the popularity of recreational activities which involve contact with water has grown. Moreover, ease of travel has altered the public use of water for recreational purposes.

Recreational exposures to pathogens in the water environment may result in disease. Susceptible populations including people with reduced immune function e.g., resulting from disease (cancer, human immunodeficiency virus (HIV), genetic susceptibility, (age etc.) or lack of acquired immunity to locally endemic diseases (e.g., tourists) may be at higher risk of contracting severe illnesses. Due to the development of protective clothing for use in colder climates, prolonged periods of contact and immersion are becoming more frequent and water-based activities occur throughout the year, not just during restricted seasons. Many infections occur on a seasonal basis and therefore users will be exposed to different and unfamiliar pathogens in the water in different locations and at different times.

The World Health Organization (WHO) has been actively involved in the protection of human health from the use of recreational waters since the 1970s. In 2003 and 2005, WHO published volumes 1 and 2 respectively of the *Guidelines for Safe Recreational Water Environments*. The Guidelines provide an assessment of the health risks associated with recreational use of water and outline linkages to monitoring and management practices. In terms of the hazards associated with recreational water activities, the *Guidelines* review the evidence accrued from epidemiological studies proving a link between gastroenteritis, acute febrile respiratory illness (AFRI), ear infections and other generally minor self-limiting illnesses and faecally-contaminated water.

In most cases the clinical conditions (or primary disease symptoms) associated with waterborne disease, including those associated with the use of water for recreational purposes, are acute, such as diarrhoea, vomiting and acute respiratory infections. Although less frequently reported and authenticated, more serious and potentially fatal disease is a risk to recreational users of water especially in certain susceptible populations. In addition to diseases which have severe primary outcomes (e.g., primary amoebic meningoencephalitis, typhoid, leptospirosis), a number of infections may lead to sequelae which are more severe than diseases commonly caused by the pathogen including renal disease (from *E. coli* O157:H7 for example), cardiac and nutritional disorders.

This publication sets out to describe the more severe waterborne diseases (and their sequelae) which may be acquired while undertaking water-based recreation in marine, freshwater, hot tubs, spas and swimming pools. The document provides the following information:

- An in-depth review of factors that lead to disease severity;
- Evidence for the frequency and severity of different types of sequelae potentially associated with diseases that can be transmitted through recreational water use;
- An extensive review of information concerning susceptible subpopulations that are particularly prone to severe diseases outcomes for specific pathogens;
- A modified classification system for establishing the credibility of disease transmission through recreational water exposures;
- An objective disease severity rating system that will facilitate the prioritization of health protection measures by public health professionals; and
- A pathogen by pathogen review that summarizes the available information on infectivity; susceptible population subgroups; environmental occurrence; evidence for disease transmission through recreational exposures; and rates the plausibility of recreational water disease transmission routes for each pathogen.

Chapters 1–3 provide the evidence for the diseases of interest, and discuss the special factors that lead to more severe disease and/or sequelae as an evaluation of disease severity. Chapters 4-6 review the evidence for severe outcomes from bacteria, protozoa/trematodes and viruses that may be encountered in recreational waters.

For the purposes of this review, the illnesses that have been considered are those where there may be a significant risk of mortality if untreated, those for which the severity of the symptoms usually requires medical intervention, and those where not all patients may recover fully but may suffer from residual symptoms which may last the rest of the patient's life. This review does not cover illnesses caused by oil, chemicals, biological toxins such as toxic cyanobacteria, or heavy metals.

This review will be useful to those concerned with recreational water quality, including environmental and public health officers, special interest groups, regulators, researchers and professionals in the fields of water supply and management of recreational water.

Acknowledgements

The World Health Organization wishes to express its appreciation to all those whose efforts made possible the production of this document, in particular to Dr. Kathy Pond (Robens Centre for Public and Environmental Health, University of Surrey, Guildford, United Kingdom) who prepared the document. Special thanks are also due to the United States Environmental Protection Agency, Office of Research and Development who provided financial support for this project.

The important contributions to this document from the following are also gratefully acknowledged:

Nicholas Ashbolt, University of New South Wales, Sydney, Australia
Jamie Bartram, WHO, Geneva, Switzerland
Edith Campbell, formerly Robens Centre for Public and Environmental Health, University of Surrey, Guildford, United Kingdom
Richard Carr, WHO, Geneva, Switzerland
Aidan Cronin, Robens Centre for Public and Environmental Health, University of Surrey, Guildford, United Kingdom
Maddalena Castellani, Istituto Superiore di Sanita, Rome, Italy

Alfred P Dufour, United States Environmental Protection Agency, Cincinnati, United States of America

Vicky Garner, formerly Surfers Against Sewage, Newquay, United Kingdom

Ann Grimm, United States Environmental Protection Agency, Cincinnati, USA

Magnea Hjálmarsdóttir, Robens Centre for Public and Environmental Health, University of Surrey, Guildford, United Kingdom

Paul Hunter, University of East Anglia, Norwich, United Kingdom

Kali Johal, Robens Centre for Public and Environmental Health, University of Surrey, Guildford, United Kingdom

David Kay, Centre for Research into Health and the Environment, University of Wales, Lampeter, United Kingdom

Gunhild Hoy Kock-Hansen, The Statens Serum Institut, Department of Epidemiology, Copenhagen, Denmark

Patricia McCusker formerly, Robens Centre for Public and Environmental Health, University of Surrey, Guildford, United Kingdom

E. Pagano, Office Fédéral de la Santé Publique, Epidémiologie et Maladies Infectieuses, Switzerland

Steve Pedley, Robens Centre for Public and Environmental Health, University of Surrey, Guildford, United Kingdom

Rosa Cano Portero, Sección de Información Microbiológica, Centro Nacional de Epidemiología, Madrid, Spain

Gareth Rees, Askham Bryan College, York, United Kingdom

Joerg Rueedi, Robens Centre for Public and Environmental Health, University of Surrey, Guildford, United Kingdom

M. Spalekova, Centre for Communicable Diseases, Institute of Public Health of the Republic of Slovenia, Trubarjeva 2, 1000 Ljublijana, Slovakia.

List of Acronyms and Abbreviations

AFRI   Acute febrile respiratory illness
AIDS   Acquired immunodeficiency syndrome
CDC   Centers for Disease Control and Prevention, USA
CDR   Communicable Disease Report
CDSC   Communicable Disease Surveillance Centre, United Kingdom
DALY   Disability-adjusted life year
DNA   Deoxyribonucleic acid
E. coli   *Escherichia coli*
EHEC   Enterohaemorrhagic *E. coli*
EU   European Union
HAV   Hepatitis A virus
HEV   Hepatitis E virus
HIV   Human immunodeficiency virus
HUS   Haemolytic uraemic syndrome
IDDM   Insulin dependent diabetes mellitus
IgG   Immunoglobulin G
MAC   *Mycobacterium avium* complex

MRA	Microbial risk assessment
PAM	Primary amoebic meningoencephalitis
PHLS	Public Health Laboratory Service, United Kingdom
QMRA	Quantitative Microbial Risk Assessment
RNA	Ribonucleic acid
SMI	Swedish Institute for Infectious Disease Control
TTP	Thrombotic thrombocytopenic purpura
US EPA	United States Environmental Protection Agency
UV	Ultraviolet
WBDO	Waterborne Disease Outbreak
WHO	World Health Organization

Executive Summary

The use of water for recreational purposes poses a number of health risks which depend on factors such as the nature of the hazard, the characteristic of the water body and the immune status of the user. Although evidence from outbreak reports and other epidemiological evidence have proven a link between adverse health effects and immersion in poor quality recreational water, the difficulties associated with attributing an infection to recreational water use are numerous and the majority of research in this field has focussed on infections associated with the use of recreational waters resulting in minor, self-limiting symptoms.

There are many unanswered questions regarding the severity and frequency of illness associated with recreational water use. It is plausible that more serious illnesses could result from the recreational use of water and this association has not yet been investigated to any great extent. It is also increasingly apparent that a number of micro-organisms or their products are directly or indirectly associated with secondary health outcomes or sequelae and a number of these sequelae may result from waterborne infections. The acute diseases attributable to waterborne pathogens and their epidemiology have been well described, but the sequelae that can result from these diseases have not. Assessing potential sequelae of waterborne infections is a critical part of microbial risk assessment and the formulation of public policy.

Even where illness is severe, it may still be difficult to attribute it to recreational water exposure due to the large number of other transmission routes of the pathogens in question. Nevertheless, evidence does exist to show that although much less frequent, more serious and potentially fatal disease is a risk to recreational users of water. This book describes the more severe waterborne diseases (and their sequelae) which may be acquired while undertaking water-based recreation in marine, freshwater, hot tubs, spas and swimming pools. A 'weight of evidence' approach has been developed to establish the credibility of association of an illness with recreational water exposure. The approach takes into account epidemiology, microbiology and water quality information. Outbreaks are therefore categorised as being 'strongly', 'probably' or 'possibly' associated with water.

Consideration of whether an illness is severe or not is based on three factors:

- acute symptoms of the disease which are debilitating;
- the ability and probability that the illness will lead to sequelae; and
- the effect of the disease on certain susceptible subpopulations.

Each factor can be considered in its own right or in combination with one or both of the other factors. A simplified index of severity has been created and applied wherever possible to the illnesses considered, taking into account possible sequelae. The outcome measures used to ascertain the relative severity are case-fatality rate, average duration of illness, median percentage of cases requiring hospitalisation, the frequency of development of sequelae and the severity of sequelae. The index is limited by the availability of data and does not take into account the probability of infection following exposure. The index is designed to help public health professionals prioritize recreational water management decisions to reduce the potential for severe disease outcomes.

The following pathogens have been considered:

Campylobacter jejuni — one of the most common causes of bacterial gastroenteritis and chronic sequelae. The pathogen has been isolated from recreational waters on many occasions. However, few cases of illness have been reported through this route. *Campylobacter jejuni* is more likely to be found in recreational waters contaminated by animal and human waste.

E. coli O157 — although most outbreaks of *E. coli* O157 have been associated with food, a number of outbreaks have been reported from recreational use of waters, particularly in pools that were not adequately chlorinated. Haemolytic uraemic syndrome with possible long-term sequelae is evident although no follow-up studies appear to have been conducted in people who contracted the infection from recreational water use. The acute disease tends to be moderately severe and of moderate duration.

Helicobacter pylori — water has been implicated as one mode of transmission of *H. pylori* although the detection of the pathogen has proved difficult. Therefore, it is possible that *H. pylori* infection is waterbome, but these assumptions need to be substantiated. Current evidence for its association with recreational waters is slight.

Legionella spp. — there are a number of reports of Legionnaires' disease associated with the use of, and proximity to, hot tubs in particular. The illness is considered to be severe with a high risk of death and severe acute symptoms. There are a number of documented cases of persons suffering sequelae as a consequence of infection with *Legionella* spp.

Mycobacterium avium complex — there is clear evidence for the association of *Mycobacterium avium* complex with recreational waters. The species of Mycobacterium that are associated with water are associated with a variety of diseases. Some, such as *M. ulverans* are pathogenic in previously healthy individuals, others, such as *M. avium*, usually cause disease in compromised individuals. The majority of cases associated with recreational waters appear to be attributed to swimming pools and hot tubs resulting in skin and soft tissue infections in immunocompetent patients. However, hypersensitivity pneumonitis is also seen in immunocompetent persons with aerosol exposure to mycobacteria.

Shigella spp. — epidemiological evidence exists for the association of recreational use of water and self-limiting infection with shigella bacteria. The species responsible for the more severe illness, *S. dysenteriae,* is more common in tropical regions but no cases associated with recreational waters were found in the literature. However, it is biologically plausible that *S. dysenteriae* could be encountered in freshwaters used for recreation.

Vibrio vulnificus — this bacteria commonly occurs in marine and estuarine environments. Evidence exists for the association of recreational use of water and infection with *V. vulnificus* where the user has a pre-existing open wound. Surveillance of *V. vulnificus* infections is poor and the number of cases reported is likely to be underestimated.

Cryptosporidium — faecal accidents are implicated in most of the cases as the cause of the outbreaks of cryptosporidiosis, which have primarily occurred in swimming pools, although some cases have been documented from water slides, fountains and water parks. *Cryptosporidium* oocysts show resistance to chlorination. The risk of death and probability of developing long-term sequelae from this infection is low, however the acute illness can be prolonged and moderately severe especially in immunocompromised persons.

Giardia — recreational use of water is a proven risk factor for giardiasis. The majority of symptomatic patients of *Giardia* will clear their infection after one to several weeks although immunocompromised patients may not recover from giardiasis. The risk of death and the probability of developing sequelae from this infection is low, however the acute illness can be prolonged and moderately severe.

Microsporidia — although microsporidia are currently not common causes of recreational waterborne disease, their role as emerging pathogens is being increasingly recognised. Their small size makes them difficult to remove by conventional water filtration techniques and it is thought that, like *Cryptosporidium* they may show increased resistance to chlorine disinfection. Illness is generally reported in immunocompromised individuals although some infections in immunocompetent individuals have been reported.

Naegeria fowleri has been shown to colonise warm freshwater habitats, such as swimming pools and natural hot springs and there is a high risk of death in infected persons. The acute illness is severe with symptoms lasting more than seven days and death always occurs. Although the infection is rare, new cases are reported every year.

Schistosoma spp. — in some cases serious pathology associated with infection by *Schistosoma spp.* occurs and can lead to long-term health issues. Schistosoma is only a potential hazard in certain geographic areas (e.g., sub-Saharan Africa). Surveillance for schistosomiasis is currently poor, inferring that many more cases associated with recreational waters occur but are not published. Evidence shows that exposure to schistosomes is difficult to avoid but it has been shown that towel-drying after exposure to infested water can markedly reduce the risk of infection.

Adenovirus — the diseases resulting from infection with adenovirus include conjunctivitis, pharyngitis, pneumonia, acute and chronic appendicitis, bronchiolitis, acute respiratory disease, and gastroenteritis. Adenovirus infections are generally mild; however, there are a number of fatal cases of infection reported in the literature. Transmission of adenovirus in recreational waters, primarily inadequately chlorinated swimming pools, has been documented via faecally-contaminated water and through droplets, although no fatal cases attributable to recreational waters have been documented in the literature.

Coxsackievirus — although there have been very few outbreaks of coxsackievirus linked to recreational water recorded, and epidemiological evidence remains scarce the virus has been frequently isolated from marine and freshwaters. As with other viruses (hepatitis A virus (HAV), adenovirus and echovirus) transmission of the virus is possible and biologically plausible in susceptible persons. Coxsackievirus is responsible for a broad range of illness from mild febrile illness to myocarditis and other more serious diseases.

Echovirus — as with the other enteroviruses discussed in this review, there are few published cases of infection by echovirus in recreational water, those that are recorded are primarily from swimming pool water. The most likely source of the virus is through faecal contamination, although secretions from the eyes or throat are possible. There are likely to be many unreported cases of infection with echovirus.

Hepatitis A virus — has been isolated from surface waters which may be used for recreational purposes and a number of cases of HAV have been documented associated with recreational water users. Fulminant hepatitis is rare and has not been reported in any cases linked with the use of recreational waters. No cases of sequelae of HAV contracted through the use of recreational waters were found in the literature and the probability of developing long-term sequelae is low. The acute disease is usually moderately severe and of moderate duration but risk of death is low.

Hepatitis E virus (HEV) — has been isolated from surface waters which may be used for recreational purposes. Fulminant hepatitis is rare. No cases of sequelae of HEV contracted through the use of recreational waters were found in the literature and the probability of developing long-term sequelae is low. The acute disease is usually moderately severe and of moderate duration but risk of death is low except where cases occur during pregnancy.

1

Introduction

1.1 BACKGROUND

Recreational use of inland and marine waters is increasing in many countries. It is estimated that foreign and local tourists together spend around two billion days annually at coastal recreational resorts (Shuval 2003). The World Tourism Organization predicts that by 2026, 346 million tourists will visit Mediterranean destinations annually, representing about 22% of all arrivals worldwide (WTO 2001). It has been estimated that 129 million people visited the beach or waterside in the United States of America between 2000 and 2001, an increase of 6% from 1995 (NOAA 2004). In the United Kingdom it is estimated that over 20 million people use the British coast each year, in addition to inland waters and their surrounding areas, for a variety of reasons. The National Centre for Social Research (1998) reported there were 241 million day visits to the sea/coast in Great Britain in 1998, with people prepared to travel an average of 43 miles to reach the coast. However, perceived risks involving recreational water use may have important economic repercussions in areas that depend to a large extent on recreational tourism as a source of income. An example is the decline in tourists visiting Lake Malawi in South Africa because of news reports about schistosomiasis cases (WHO 2003a).

Indoor water recreation is also hugely popular. Pools may be private (domestic), semi-public (hotels, schools, health clubs, cruise ships) or public (municipal or governmental). Pools may be supplied with fresh, marine or thermal water. Specialist pools, such as hot tubs are used for both pleasure and medicinal purposes and are generally filled with water at temperatures over 32°C (WHO 2005). 'Natural spa' is the term used to refer to facilities containing thermal and/or mineral water, some of which may be perceived to have therapeutic value and, because of certain water characteristics, may receive minimal water treatment (WHO 2005).

Water-based recreation and tourism can expose individuals to a variety of health hazards, including pathogenic micro-organisms. Sports which involve intimate contact with the water such as surfing, windsurfing and scuba diving are growing in popularity, and technology is changing the behaviour of recreational water users – the use of wet suits for example, now encouraging prolonged immersion in water even in temperate or cool areas. The type, design and use of pools may predispose the user to certain hazards. Indoor pools, for example, may be subject to higher bather-loads relative to the volume of water. Where there are high water temperatures and rapid agitation of water, it may become difficult to maintain microbiological quality, adequate disinfectant residual and a satisfactory pH (WHO 2005).

The vast majority of research to date in the field of recreational water quality and health has focused on microbial hazards, in particular gastroenteric outcomes arising from contamination of water by sewage and excreta. Mild gastroenteric symptoms are widespread and common amongst recreational water users. A cause-effect relationship between bather-derived pollution or faecal pollution and acute febrile respiratory illness (AFRI) is biologically plausible, and a significant exposure-response relationship (between AFRI and faecal streptococci) has been reported by Fleisher *et al.* (1996). AFRI is a more severe health outcome than self-limiting gastrointestinal symptoms, but probabilities of contracting AFRI are generally lower and the threshold at which the illness is observed is higher (WHO 2003a).

Despite the acknowledged constraints of current bathing water quality monitoring practices, considerable information has become available to recreational water users in recent years concerning the microbial quality of the water they are using for recreation. The relatively minor illnesses associated with poor microbial quality of water and non-microbial hazards have been identified in the WHO *Guidelines for Safe Recreational Water Environments* (WHO 2003a; WHO 2005). Less information is available on the more severe potential health outcomes encountered by recreational water users resulting in symptoms which are not self-limiting and require medical attention.

Waterborne microbial pathogens are capable of causing illness depending on the dose and the physical condition of the individuals exposed. It should be stressed that exposure to waterborne pathogens does not always result in infection[1], nor does infection always lead to clinical illness.

The total global health impact of human infectious diseases associated with pathogenic micro-organisms from land-based wastewater pollution of coastal areas has been estimated at about three million disability-adjusted life years (DALYs) per year, with an estimated economic loss of around 12 billion dollars per year (Shuval 2003).

Researchers in the United States have estimated that the health burden of swimming-related illnesses at two popular beaches in California, USA exceeds US $3.3 million per year. The annual costs for each type of swimming-related illness at the two beaches were estimated to be: gastrointestinal illnesses, US $1,345,339; acute respiratory disease, US $951,378; ear complaints, US $767,221; eye complaints, US $304,335 (Dwight et al. 2005).

Although most illnesses contracted through recreational water contact are mild (e.g., self-limiting diarrhoea) diseases with a range of severities may also occur. A number of viruses, bacteria and protozoa associated with more severe health outcomes may plausibly be transmitted through use of contaminated recreational water. Bacteria and protozoa may induce illnesses with a wide range of severity. Bacteria may cause life-threatening diseases such as typhoid, cholera and leptospirosis. Viruses can cause serious diseases such as aseptic meningitis, encephalitis, poliomyelitis, hepatitis, myocarditis and diabetes. Protozoa may cause primary amoebic meningoencephalitis (PAM) and schistosomiasis is caused by a flatworm (trematode). In addition, gastrointestinal disorders are amongst a number of illnesses that may be attributed to unidentified or unspecified micro-organisms.

These hazards to human health should be weighed against the benefits of using water as a medium for relaxation and aerobic, non-weight bearing exercise. Physical exercise has been shown to positively affect certain cardiovascular risk factors such as insulin resistance, glucose metabolism, blood pressure and body fat composition, which are closely associated with diabetes and heart disease. With increasingly sedentary life styles in many societies, routine daily exercise of moderate intensity is highly recommended to reduce cardiovascular risk (Li et al. 2003). Swimming is often recommended by the medical profession because of its potentially beneficial effect on the joints and indeed on people's general sense of well-being. For example, non-swimming dynamic exercises in heated water have been shown to have a positive impact on individuals with late effects of polio, with a decreased heart rate at exercise, less pain, and a subjective positive experience (Willen et al. 2001). Although it

---

[1] Infection - The initial entry of a pathogen into a host; the condition in which a pathogen has become established in or on the cells or tissues of a host. Such a condition does not necessarily constitute or lead to a disease (Singleton and Sainsbury 2001).

is difficult to quantify the psychological benefits of exercise, Van de Vliet *et al.* (2004) have shown that fitness training embedded in a cognitive-behavioural treatment programme is associated with positive changes in clinically depressed patients. This includes enhanced coping strategies, sustained efforts to continue activities, and improved awareness of physical well-being.

1.2 EVIDENCE FOR ADVERSE HEALTH OUTCOMES ASSOCIATED WITH RECREATIONAL WATER USE

The first reviews of the incidence of disease associated with the use of recreational waters were undertaken by the American Public Health Association in the early 1920s. Simons *et al.* (1922) attempted to determine the prevalence of infectious diseases which may be transmitted by recreational water contact.

Major epidemiological studies were conducted between 1948 and 1950 by the United States Public Health Service (Stevenson 1953) to investigate the link between bathing and illness. The findings concluded that there was an appreciably higher overall illness incidence rate in people who swam in Lake Michigan, Chicago, the United States, in 1948 and on the Ohio River at Dayton, Kentucky, the United States, in 1949 compared with non-swimmers, regardless of the levels of coliform bacteria found in the water quality tests. It was concluded by Stevenson (1953) that, based upon the results of this study, the stricter bacterial quality requirements could be relaxed without a detrimental effect on the health of bathers.

Moore (1959) undertook a similar study in the United Kingdom. His study was based on five years of investigation of 43 beaches in the United Kingdom and concluded that there was only a 'negligible risk to health' of bathing in sewage polluted sea water even when beaches were 'aesthetically very unsatisfactory' and that a serious risk would only exist if the water was so fouled as to be revolting to the senses. Moore insisted that pathogenic bacteria which were isolated from sewage contaminated sea water were more important as indicators of the disease in the population than as evidence of a health risk in the waters.

The subject became one of controversy for many years. It was acknowledged in 1972 by the United States Environmental Protection Agency (US EPA) that there was a lack of valid epidemiological data with which to set guideline standards for recreational waters. There followed a number of epidemiological studies throughout the world (Table 1.1). In many of the studies identified in Table 1.1, the occurrence of certain symptoms or symptom groups was found to be significantly related to the count of faecal indicator bacteria or bacterial pathogens. Credible associations were found between gastrointestinal symptoms (including 'highly credible' or 'objective' symptoms) and indicators such as enterococci, faecal streptococci, thermotolerant coliforms and *E. coli*.

The WHO *Guidelines for Safe Recreational Water Environments* reviewed the scientific evidence concerning the health issues associated with using waters for recreational purposes and concluded that enteric illness, such as self-limiting gastroenteritis, and AFRI are the most frequently investigated and reported adverse health outcomes in the published literature. The *Guidelines* also concluded that there is an association between gastrointestinal symptoms, AFRI and indicator-bacteria concentrations in recreational waters (WHO 2003a; WHO 2005). The *Guidelines* represent a consensus view and assessment among experts of the health hazards encountered during recreational water use. It includes the derivation of guideline values and explains the basis for the decision to derive or not to derive them.

There are relatively few studies which report associations between indicators and other symptoms although there is limited evidence of an association between ear (Fleisher *et al.* 1996), eye (Fleisher *et al.* 1996) and skin ailments with swimming. Evidence suggests that bathing, regardless of water quality, compromises the eye's immune defences leading to increased reporting of symptoms after bathing in marine waters. Infection could also be due to person-to-person transmission (Hunter 1998). In addition, the statistical probability of contracting an ear infection has been found to be generally lower than for gastrointestinal illnesses which are associated with higher thermotolerant coliform concentrations (WHO 2003a). Several studies have found that symptom rates were more frequent in lower age groups (Cabelli 1983; Fattal *et al.* 1987; UNEP/WHO 1991; Pike 1994).

As illustrated in Table 1.1, the main focus of effort concerning the health implications of the recreational use of water focuses on the effects of faecal contamination of bathing waters and the incidence of gastrointestinal diseases and other transmissible diseases to participants in water recreation. The data concerning some of the other hazards is weaker. There are very few epidemiological studies which have considered special interest activities (Table 1.2). Evans *et al.* (1983) found no evidence of any particular health risk from short-term immersion in Bristol City Docks, UK. However, Philipp *et al.* (1985) studied the health of snorkel swimmers in the same body of water who were immersed for 40 minutes and revealed that statistically significantly more swimmers reported gastrointestinal symptoms compared with the control group, even though the water complied with the European Union (EU) bathing water standards.

Medema *et al.* (1995) investigating the risk of gastroenteritis in triathlete swimmers estimated that the exposure of triathletes during a competition was between 15 and 40 minutes and exposure was relatively intense; 75% of all triathletes in his study were comapred with biathletes and it was reported that although the health risks for triathletes were not significantly higher than for run-bike-runners (biathletes) symptoms were higher in the week after the event in those athletes that had been exposed to water.

Table 1.1 Major epidemiological studies investigating the health effects from exposure to recreational water conducted between 1953 and 1996 (Adapted from Prüss 1998).

First author	Year	Country	Type of water
Fleisher*	1996	United Kingdom	Marine
Haile*	1996	United States	Marine
Van Dijk	1996	United Kingdom	Marine
Van Asperen	1995	The Netherlands	Fresh
Bandaranayake*	1995	New Zealand	Marine
Kueh*	1995	China	Marine
Medical Research Council*	1995	South Africa	Marine
Kay*	1994	United Kingdom	Marine
Pike*	1994	United Kingdom	Marine
Fewtrell	1994	United Kingdom	Fresh
Von Schirnding	1993	South Africa	Marine
McBride	1993	New Zealand	Marine
Corbett	1993	Australia	Marine
Harrington	1993	Australia	Marine
Von Schirnding	1992	South Africa	Marine
Fewtrell*	1992	United Kingdom	Fresh
Alexander	1991	United Kingdom	Marine
Jones	1991	United Kingdom	Marine
Balarajan	1991	United Kingdom	Marine
UNEP/WHO*	1991	Israel	Marine
UNEP/WHO*	1991	Spain	Marine
Cheung*	1990	China	Marine
Ferley*	1989	France	Fresh
Lightfoot	1989	Canada	Fresh
New Jersey Department of Health	1989	United States	Marine
Brown	1987	United Kingdom	Marine
Fattal, UNEP/WHO*	1987	Israel	Marine
Philipp	1985	United Kingdom	Fresh
Seyfried*	1985	Canada	Fresh
Dufour*	1984	United States	Fresh
Foulon	1983	France	Marine
Cabelli*	1983	Egypt	Marine
El Sharkawi	1982	Egypt	Marine
Calderon	1982	United States	Marine
Cabelli*	1982	United States	Fresh and Marine
Mujeriego*	1982	Spain	Marine
Public Health Laboratory Service	1959	United Kingdom	Marine
Stevenson*	1953	United States	Fresh and Marine

*indicates the rate of certain symptoms or symptom group was found to be significantly related to the count of faecal indicator bacteria or bacterial pathogen.

The results of the study of van Asperen (1998) were consistent with that of Medema *et al.* (1997). The study showed that of those who reported swallowing water during the swimming period reported gastroenteritis more frequently

(6.8%) than those that did not (3.8%). The percentage of triathletes swallowing water was 72%.

Dwight *et al.* (2004) compared rates of reported health symptoms among surfers during two winters. Their findings showed that for every 2.5 hours of weekly water exposure, surfers experienced a 10% increase in probability of illness (a variety of different symptoms were tracked including highly credible gastrointestinal illness, stomach pain, vomiting, diarrhoea, and others).

These activities are important to consider since the difference in risk between the various uses of recreational waters lies primarily with the duration of exposure and the quantity of water ingested.

Different behaviours of different populations of swimmers are an important risk factor for infection. For example, swimming in unchlorinated open waters is much more common in warmer climates and this may increase the risk of illness to swimmers.

For several reasons, children are at particular risk of contracting recreational waterborne illness. Children have greater opportunities for exposure; they tend to be more frequent users of recreational waters for longer periods of time compared to older age groups, and their activities, which may involve play, often increase exposure to contaminated water through accidental ingestion.

Table 1.2 Epidemiological studies considering water activities other than bathing (Environment Agency, England and Wales 2002; Dwight *et al.* 2004)

First author	Date	Activity	Country	Type of water
Dwight	2004	Surfers	USA	Marine
Van Asperen	1998	Triathlon	The Netherlands	Freshwater
Gammie	1997	Surfers/windsurfers	United Kingdom	Marine and freshwater
Lee	1997	White-water canoeing	United Kingdom	Freshwater
Medema	1995	Triathlon	The Netherlands	Freshwater
Fewtrell	1994	Rowing and marathon canoeing	United Kingdom	Freshwater canals and estuaries
Fewtrell	1992	White-water canoeing	United Kingdom	Freshwater
Philipp	1985	Snorkelling	United Kingdom	Freshwater docks
Evans	1983	Variety of water sports	United Kingdom	Freshwater docks

Figure 1.1 shows the outbreaks of disease associated with recreational water contact reported to the United States CDC between 1978 and 2002. The data indicate that reported gastroenteritis outbreaks related to recreational water use are increasing in the USA. Although not directly comparable, Galbraith *et al.* (1987) reported relatively few outbreaks associated with recreational water use in the United Kingdom between 1937 and 1986.

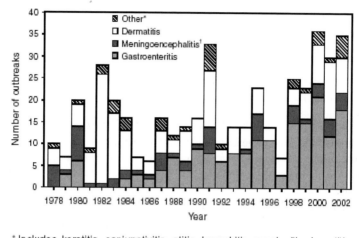

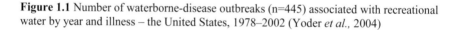

* Includes keratitis, conjunctivitis, otitis, bronchitis, meningitis, hepatitis, leptospirosis, Pontiac fever, and acute respiratory illness.
† Also includes data from report of ameba infections (Source: Visvesvara GS, Stehr-Green JK. Epidemiology of free-living ameba infections. J Protozool 1990;37:25S–33S).

Figure 1.1 Number of waterborne-disease outbreaks (n=445) associated with recreational water by year and illness – the United States, 1978–2002 (Yoder *et al.*, 2004)

The documented health risks posed by poor quality bathing waters usually relate to acute infections acquired whilst bathing. Most of the epidemiological studies conducted to establish a link between bathing and illness do not address the more severe health outcomes or possible sequelae. This is probably due to the low occurrence of severe health outcomes in recent decades in the temperate regions where the majority of studies have been conducted, and because investigations of rarer outcomes usually require larger study groups.

1.3 SEVERE OUTCOMES

For the purposes of this review, consideration of whether an illness is severe or not is based on three factors:
- acute symptoms of the disease which are debilitating;
- the ability and probability that the illness will lead to sequelae; and
- the effect of the disease on certain susceptible subpopulations.

Each factor can be considered in its own right or in combination with one or both of the other factors.

WHO microbial guideline values for safe recreational water environments are in fact based on evidence of the transmission of relatively mild gastrointestinal illness and AFRI. However, the guidelines make provision for adjustment where there is more severe disease plausibly associated with recreational water use circulating in the population. The use of DALYs is suggested as a useful approach to do this. Management approaches developed in the WHO *Guidelines* when implemented as suggested will help to mitigate both mild and severe infectious illnesses transmitted through recreational water.

1.3.1 Infections with potentially severe acute symptoms

Although the majority of illnesses transmitted through recreational water use are relatively mild and often self-limiting, there are a number of waterborne pathogens that can cause illnesses with severe outcomes even in average populations.

These include: *Campylobacter* spp., *E. coli* O157, *Salmonella typhi*, *Shigella* spp., *Leptospira icterohaemorrhagiae*, HAV, *Cryptosporidium parvum* and a number of others described throughout this review. Some of these have been known for many years; others, such as *Helicobacter pylori*, are emerging as new pathogens or re-emerging after many years (WHO 2003b). Although not always severe, infection by these pathogens can result in hospitalisation, surgery and death. For example, leptospirosis has been found to have a case-fatality rate as high as 22% if left untreated (Ciceroni *et al.* 2000) and a hospitalisation rate of 30–50% (Smythe *et al.* 2000; Sasaki *et al.* 1993). The primary disease symptoms caused by infections with these pathogens are shown in Table 1.3.

1.3.2 Evidence for sequelae of waterborne diseases

Sequelae are increasingly important to food and drinking-water risk assessment. It has been estimated that around 5% of waterborne diseases result in sequelae (Reynolds 2003). There has been little agreement over a scientific definition for sequelae. The Oxford English Dictionary defines a sequela as 'a morbid affection occurring as a result of previous disease' (Weiner and Simpson 1989). Parkin *et al.* (2000) reviewed scientific publications for definitions of chronic sequelae and developed a definition as follows:

'the secondary health outcome that (1) occurs as a result of a previous infection by a microbial pathogen; (2) is clearly distinguishable from the health events that initially result from the causative infection and (3) lasts three months or more after recognition'.

Table 1.3 Pathogens that may cause severe acute disease outcomes

Pathogen	Primary disease symptoms
Campylobacter spp.	Diarrhoea, occasionally bloody and severe. Cramping abdominal pain, fever, malaise.
Salmonella typhi	Typhoid – fever, malaise, aches, abdominal pain, diarrhoea or constipation, delirium.
Shigella dysenteriae	Severe abdominal pain, watery diarrhoea or stools containing blood.
Leptospira spp.	High fever, severe headache, chills, muscle aches, and vomiting, and may include jaundice (yellow skin and eyes), red eyes, abdominal pain, diarrhoea, or a rash.
Giardia spp.	Acute onset of diarrhoea, abdominal cramps, bloating and flatulence, malaise, weight loss.
E. coli O157:H7	Severe bloody diarrhoea and abdominal cramps; sometimes the infection causes non-bloody diarrhoea or no symptoms.
Cryptosporidium spp.	Diarrhoea, mild abdominal pain, mild fever.
Viral hepatitis - hepatitis A and E	Malaise, lassitude, myalgia, arthralgia, fever and sometimes jaundice.
Helicobacter pylori	Nausea, abdominal pain, gastritis, hypochlorhydria.
Schistosomes	Itchy papular rash, other symptoms depend on the organ that the organism resides in.
Naegleria fowleri	Severe headache, fever, vomiting, neck stiffness.
Legionella spp.	Fever, cough, prostration, diarrhoea, pleuritic pain.

The sequelae symptoms may be completely different from the symptoms of the acute illness and may occur even if the immune system successfully manages to eliminate the primary infection. The action of the immune system may initiate the condition as a result of an autoimmune response (Archer and Young 1988; Bunning 1994; Bunning *et al.* 1997). However, it is also possible that the initial infection may not have passed when the secondary symptoms appear. For the purposes of this review, sequelae which may last less than three months are also included and, therefore, according to Parkin's definition (Parkin 2000) are not chronic.

The evidence that micro-organisms or their products are directly or indirectly associated with sequelae ranges from convincing to circumstantial, due to the fact that it is unlikely that such complications are identified or epidemiologically linked to the initial illness because the data are not systematically collected. In addition, host symptoms caused by a specific pathogen or product of a pathogen are often wide-ranging and difficult to link with a specific incident, particularly as the time of onset of sequelae may vary.

Table 1.4 Sequelae associated with micro-organisms found in recreational waters

Organism	Sequelae	Reference
Salmonella spp.	Septic arthritis, Reiter's syndrome	Hill *et al.* 2003
	Pyogenic lesions	Yu and Thompson 1994
	Intracranial abscess	Hanel *et al.* 2000
	Osteomyelitis	Declercq *et al.* 1994
Campylobacter spp.	Guillain-Barré syndrome	Nachamkin 2002
	Acute motor neuropathy	Wirguin *et al.* 1997
	Opthalmoplegia	Kuroki *et al.* 2001
	Reiter's syndrome	McDonald and Gruslin 2001
	Infection of various organs and the blood stream	Ang *et al.* 2001
Shigella dysenteriae	Aseptic or reactive arthritis,	Hill *et al.* 2003
	Fulminating encephalopathy	Dieu-Osika *et al.* 1996
S. flexneri	Reiter's syndrome	Van Bohemen *et al.* 1986
Giardia duodenalis	Inflammatory arthritis	Gaston Hill and Lillicrap 2003
	Disaccharide intolerance	Lane and Lloyd 2002
	Malabsorption	Hunter 1998
Mycobacterium avium complex	Tentative Crohn's disease and ulcerative colitis	Chiodini 1989
	Sarcoidosis	Li *et al.* 1999
	Osteomyelitis	Chan *et al.* 2001
E. coli O157:H7	Haemolytic uraemic syndrome	Mead and Griffin 1998
	Thrombotic thromocytopenic purpura	Kuntz and Kuntz 1999
Schistosoma spp.	Bladder cancer	WHO 1994
	Kidney disease	Rocha *et al.* 1976
	Hepatic coma	
Naegleria fowleri	Cardiac abnormalities, convulsions, lethargy	Martinez 1993
Hepatitis A	Idiopathic autoimmune chronic active hepatitis	Rahyaman *et al.* 1994
Helicobacter pylori	Acute gastritis leading to gastric mucosal atrophy, intestinal metaplasia and gastric cancer	Kuipers *et al.* 1995; 2003
Leptospira spp.	Headache, ophthalmic sequelae	Torre *et al.* 1994
	Acalculous cholecystitis, pancreatitis, hypermylasemia	Casella and Scatena 2000
	Antiphospholipid syndrome	Tattevin *et al.* 2003
Cryptosporidium spp.	Loss of fluids, anorexia, malabsorption of nutrients	Jokipii *et al.* 1983
	Shortfalls in linear growth and weight gain	Kosek *et al.* 2001
Legionella spp.	Pericarditis, respiratory failure, arthritis, seizures	Puelo Fadi *et al.* 1995
	Pancreatitis and liver abscesses	Nguyen *et al.* 1991
	Thrombocytopenia	Larsson *et al.* 1999
	Cerebral abscess	Michel *et al.* 1996

Typically, for example, if symptoms of Reiter's syndrome (reactive arthritis) appear then it will be one to three weeks after initial infection with *Salmonella* spp. Symptoms of haemolytic uraemic syndrome (HUS), if they are to appear, are usually seen within 15 days of infection with *E. coli* O157:H7. However, sequelae such as hypertension and renal failure may not manifest themselves until 15 years later (Loirat 2001). Leptospires, the bacteria causing leptospirosis, may persist in the brain — in one report, 4 out of 11 patients had persistent headaches for between 6 and 34 years post-infection; ophthalmic involvement with blurred vision has been reported to persist for decades following acute infection (Shpilberg *et al.* 1990). Where there is a long time-period between the initial symptoms and the sequelae, it becomes more difficult to prove an association between the initial disease and the delayed sequelae.

Table 1.4 provides a summary of sequelae associated with some micro-organisms which may be found in recreational waters. These will be discussed in more detail throughout this review. It is stressed that the development of a sequela is incidental to exposure to recreational water, i.e. the sequelae described in this section result from infection with certain pathogens.

Lindsay (1997) raises a further issue which is not widely discussed in the literature: the effect of chronic disease on human personality factors as a result of symptoms such as continual pain from arthritis, irritable bowel or other conditions such as chronic diarrhoea. However, these will not be discussed in this review.

1.3.3 Severe outcomes in special populations

Diseases that are normally mild and self-limiting in the general population can have severe manifestations in susceptible sub-populations with certain attributes. A variety of host factors impact susceptibility to severe disease outcomes. Human immune status can be affected by diseases (HIV, cancer), age, medications taken (e.g., chemotherapy treatment of cancer weakens the immune system), pregnancy, nutritional status, genetics and other factors (Carr and Bartram 2004). Host factors can influence both the severity of the acute symptoms and the propensity to develop sequelae (Reynolds 2003).

The population of immunocompromised individuals is growing (Soldatou and Davies 2003). This population is more susceptible to waterborne infections and tend to experience more severe outcomes (e.g., debilitating illness, death) following infection (Reynolds 2003). A number of studies have shown that enteric diseases are the most common and serious problems that affect persons with acquired immunodeficiency syndrome (AIDS). Between 50% and 90% of people with HIV/AIDS suffer from chronic diarrhoeal illness, and the effects can be fatal (Janoff and Smith 1988). People with reduced immune function due to cancer treatment have been shown to have a case-fatality rate for adenovirus infection of 53% (Hierholzer 1992). Likewise, in the 1993 *Cryptosporidium* outbreak in Milwaukee, Wisconsin, USA, 85% of the deaths occurred in people with HIV/AIDS (Hoxie *et al.* 1997). People with liver diseases are at particularly high risk of fatal septicaemia after ingestion of, or percutaneous exposure to, *Vibrio vulnificus* (Levine and Griffin 1993).

Table 1.5 shows the case-fatality observed for enteric pathogens in nursing home patients in the USA who are more susceptible to infection compared with the general population.

Table 1.5 Case-fatality observed for enteric pathogens in nursing homes compared to the general population (Adapted from Gerba *et al.* 1996)

Organism	Case-fatality (%) in general population	Case-fatality (%) in nursing home patients
Campylobacter jejuni	0.1	1.1
E. coli O157:H7	0.2	11.8
Salmonella spp.	0.1	3.8

1.4 MANAGEMENT OF SEVERE ILLNESSES

The possible adverse health outcomes associated with recreational water result in the need for guidelines that can be converted into locally appropriate standards and associated management of sites to ensure a safe, healthy and aesthetically pleasing environment (WHO 2003a). The management interventions that may be required to ensure a safe recreational water environment are outside the scope of this publication but include compliance and enforcement measures, water quality monitoring, sanitary surveys, animal waste control measures, wastewater treatment, risk communication and information dissemination to increase public awareness. The reader is referred to the WHO *Guidelines for Safe Recreational Water Environments, Volumes 1 and 2* (WHO 2003a; 2005) which illustrates how this can be best achieved through an integrated framework for assessment and management of risk for water-related infectious diseases (Kay *et al.* 2004).

1.5 SUMMARY

There are many unanswered questions regarding the severity and frequency of illness associated with recreational water use. The difficulties associated with attributing an infection to recreational water use are numerous and the majority of research in this field has focussed on infections associated with the use of recreational waters resulting in minor, self-limiting symptoms. However, it is plausible that more serious illnesses could result from the recreational use of water and this association has not yet been investigated to any great extent. It is also increasingly apparent that a number of micro-organisms or their products are directly or indirectly associated with secondary health outcomes or sequelae and a number of these sequelae may result from waterborne infections. The acute diseases attributable to waterborne pathogens and their epidemiology have been well described, but the sequelae that can result from these diseases have not. Assessing potential sequelae of waterborne infections is a critical part of microbial risk assessment and the formulation of public policy.

1.6 DOCUMENT OVERVIEW

This review identifies those micro-organisms which may be present in recreational waters and may result in more severe effects resulting from infection. Chapter 2 looks at hazard identification and quantification in recreational waters. Chapter 3 develops a framework for associating disease outcomes with recreational water exposures and presents a systematic method for ranking severity. Chapters 4–6 describe information on specific bacterial, protozoan, trematode and viral pathogens and uses the criteria outlined in Chapter 3 to establish the credibility of association for transmission of each pathogen through recreational water use.

REFERENCES

Alexander, L.M. and Heaven, A. (1991) *Health risks associated with exposure to seawater contaminated with sewage: the Blackpool Beach survey 1990,* Environmental Epidemiology Research Unit, Lancaster University, Lancaster, UK, 67pp.

Ang, C.W., De Klerk, M.A., Endtz, H.P., Jacobs, B.C., Laman, J.D., van der Meche, F.G. and van Doorn, P.A. (2001) Guillain-Barré syndrome and Miller Fisher syndrome-associated *C. jejuni* lipopolysaccharides induce anti-GM1 and anti-GQ1b antibodies in rabbits. *Infection and Immunity,* **69**(4), 2462–2469.

Archer, D.L. and Young, F.E. (1988) Contemporary issues: diseases with a food vector. *Clinical Microbiology Reviews,* **1**, 377–398.

Balarajan, R., Soni Raleigh, V., Yuen, P., Wheeler, D., Machin, D. and Cartwright, R. (1991) Health risks associated with bathing in sea water. *British Medical Journal,* **303**, 1444–1445.

Bandaranayake, D., Salmond, C., Turner, S.J., McBride, G.B., Lewis, G.D. and Till, D.G. (1995) Health effects of bathing at selected New Zealand marine beaches. Ministry for the Environment report, Auckland. 98pp.

Brown, J.M., Campbell, E.A., Riskards, A.D. and Wheeler, D. (1987) Sewage pollution of bathing water. *Lancet,* **ii**, 1208–1209.

Bunning, V.K. (1994) Immunopathogenic aspects of foodborne microbial disease. *Food Microbiology,* **11**, 89–95.

Bunning, V.K., Lindsay, J.A. and Archer, D.L. (1997) Chronic health effects of food-borne microbial disease. *World Health Statistics Quarterly,* **50**, 51–56.

Cabelli, V.J., Dufour, A.P., McCabe, L.J. and Levin, M.A. (1982) Swimming-associated gastroenteritis and water quality. *American Journal of Epidemiology,* **115**, 606–616.

Cabelli, V.J. (1983) Health effects criteria for marine recreational waters. EPA-600/11-80-031, US Environmental Protection Agency, Cincinnati, USA.

Calderon, R. and Mood, E. (1982) An epidemiological assessment of water quality and swimmers ear. *Archives of Environmental Health*, **37**, 300–305.

Carr, R. and Bartram, J. (2004) The control envelope and risk management (Chapter 5). In: Cotruvo, J.A., Dufour, A., Rees, G., Bartram, J., Carr, R., Cliver, D.O., Craun, G.F., Fayer, R., and Gannon, V.P.J. (eds.) *Waterborne Zoonoses: Identification, Causes and Control.* Published on behalf of the World Health Organization by IWA Publishing, London.

Casella, G. and Florio Scatena, L. (2000) Mild pancreatitis in leptospirosis infection. *The American Journal of Gastroenterology,* **95**(7), 1843–1844

Chan, E.D., Kong, P.M., Fennelly, K., Dwyer, A.P. and Iseman, M.D. (2001) Vertebral osteomyelitis due to infection with nontuberculous Mycobacterium species after blunt trauma to the back: 3 examples of the principle of locus minoris resistentiae. *Clinical Infectious Diseases*, **32**, 1506–1510.

Cheung, W.H.S., Chang, K.C.K. and Hung, R.P.S. (1990) Health effects of beach water pollution in Hong Kong. *Epidemiology and Infection,* **105**, 139–162.

Chiodini, R.J. (1989) Crohn's disease and the mycobacterioses: a review and comparison of two disease entities. *Clinical Microbiology Reviews*, **2**(1), 90–117.

Ciceroni, L., Stepan, E., Pinto, A., Pizzocaro, P., Dettori, G., Franzin, L., Lu Mansueto, S., Manera, A., Ioli, A., Marcuccio, L., Grillo, R. and Ciarrocchi, S. (2000) Epidemiological trend of human leptospirosis in Italy between 1994 and 1996. *European Journal of Epidemiology*, **16**(1), 79– 86.

Corbett, S.J., Rubin, G.L., Curry, G.K., Kleinbaum, D.G. (1993) The health effects of swimming at Sydney beaches. The Sydney Beach Users Advisory Group. *American Journal of Public Health,* **83**, 1701–1706.

Declercq, J., Verhaegen, J., Verbist, L., Lammens, J., Stuyck, J. and Fabry, G. (1994). *Salmonella typhi* osteomyelitis. *Archives of Orthopaedic and Trauma Surgery*, **113**, 232–234.

Dieu-Osika, S., Tazarourte-Pinturier, M.F., Dessemme, P., Rousseau, R., Sauvion, S., Nathanson, M. and Gaudelus, J. (1996) Encéphalopathie fulminante à *Shigella flexneri*. *Archives de Pédiatrie*, **3**(10), 993–996.

Dufour, A.P. (1984) Health effects criteria for fresh recreational waters. EPA 600/1–84–004, US Environmental Protection Agency, Cincinatti, Ohio 45268.

Dwight, R.H., Baker, D.B., Semenza, J.C. and Olson, B.H. (2004) Health effects associated with recreational coastal water use: urban versus rural California. *American Journal of Public Health,* **94**(4), 565–567.

Dwight, R.H., Fernandez, L.M., Baker, D.B., Semenza, J.C. and Olson, B.H. (2005) Estimating the economic burden from illnesses associated with recreational water pollution — a case study in Orange County, California. *Journal of Environmental Management,* **76**(2), 95–103.

El Sharkawi, F. and Hassan, M.N.E.R. (1982) The relation between the state of pollution in Alexandria swimming beaches and the occurrence of typhoid among bathers. *Bulletin of the High Institute of Public Health Alexandria,* **12**, 337–351.

Environment Agency, England and Wales (2002) Recreational water quality objectives and standards: Phase 1 – data collection, presentation and recommendations. *Research & Development Technical Report* P2-253/TR. Bristol, United Kingdom.

Evans, E.J., Philipp, R. and Enticott, R.G. (1983) *Survey of the health consequences of participating in water-based events in the Bristol City Docks, January 1983.* A report from the control of infection unit, Bristol and Weston Health Authority, to the Bristol City Docks Water Quality Study Group. Bristol, United Kingdom.

Fattal, B., Peleg-Olevsky, E., Agurshy, T. and Shuval, H.I. (1987) The association between sea water pollution as measured by bacterial indicators and morbidity of bathers at Mediterranean beaches in Israel. *Chemosphere*, **16**, 565–570.

Ferley, J.P., Zmirou, D., Balducci, F., Baleux, B., Fera, P., Larbaigt, G., Jacq, E., Moissonnier, B., Blineau, A. and Boudot, J. (1989) Epidemiological significance of microbiological pollution criteria for river recreational waters. *International Journal of Epidemiology*, **18**, 198–205.

Fewtrell, L., Jones, F., Kay, D., Wyer, M.D., Godfree, A.F. and Salmon, B.L. (1992) Health effects of white-water canoeing. *The Lancet*, **339**(8809), 1587–1589

Fewtrell, L., Kay, D., Salmon, R.L., Wyer, M.D., Newman, G. and Bowering, G. (1994) The health effects of low-contact water activities in fresh and estuarine waters. *Journal of the Institution of Water and Environmental Management*, **8**, 97–101.

Fleisher, J.M., Kay, D., Salmon, R.L., Jones, F., Wyer, M.D. and Godfree, A.F. (1996) Marine waters contaminated with domestic sewage: nonenteric illness associated with bather exposure in the United Kingdom. *American Journal of Public Health*, **86**, 1228–1234.

Foulon, G., Maurin, J., Quoi, N.N., Martin-Bouyer, G. (1983) Etude de la morbidité humaine en relation avec la pollution bactériolgique des eaux de baignade en mer. *Revue Française des Sciences de l'Eau*, **2**, 127–143.

Galbraith, N.S., Barrett, N.J. and Stanwell-Smith, R. (1987) Water and disease after Croydon: a review of water-borne and water-associated disease in the UK 1937–1986. *Journal of the Institution of Water and Environmental Management*, **1**, 7–21.

Gammie, A.J. and Wyn-Jones, A.P. (1997) Does Hepatitis A pose a significant health risk to recreational water users? *Water Science and Technology*, **35**(11–12), 171–177.

Gaston Hill, J.S. and Lillicrap, M.S. (2003) Arthritis associated with enteric infection. *Best Practice & Research in Clinical Rheumatology*, **17**(2), 219–239.

Gerba, C.P., Rose, J.B. and Haas, C.N. (1996) Sensitive populations: who is at the greatest risk? *International Journal of Food Microbiology*, **30**, 113–123.

Haile, W. (1996) *An epidemiological study of possible health effects of swimming in Santa Monica Bay*. Final Report. Santa Monica Bay Restoration Project, California.

Harrington, J.F., Wilcox, D.N., Giles, P.S., Ashbolt, N.J., Evans, J.C. and Kirton, H.C. (1993) The health of Sydney surfers: an epidemiological study. *Water Science and Technology*, 27(3-4), 175–181.

Hanel, R.A., Araújo, J.C., Antoniuk, A., da Silva Ditzel, F.L., Terezinha, L., Martins, F. and Linhares, M.N. (2000) Multiple brain abscesses caused by *Salmonella typhi*: case report. *Surgical Neurology*, **53**(1), 86–90.

Hierholzer, J.C. (1992) Adenovirus in the immunocompromised host. *Clinics in Microbiological Reviews*, **5**, 262–274.

Hill, J.S., Gaston, M. and Lillicrap, S. (2003) Arthritis associated with enteric infection. *Best Practice & Research Clinical Rheumatology*, **17** (2), 219–239.

Hoxie, N.J., Davis, J.P., Vergeront, J.M., Nashold, R.D., Blair, K.A. (1997). Cryptosporidiosis-associated mortality following a massive waterborne outbreak in Milwaukee, Wisconsin. *American Journal of Public Health*, **87**(12), 2032–2035.

Hunter, P. (1998) *Waterborne Disease. Epidemiology and Ecology*. John Wiley and Sons Ltd, Chichester, UK, New York, USA.

Janoff, E.D. and Smith, P.D. (1988) Perspectives on gastrointestinal infections in AIDS. *Gastroenterology Clinics of North America*, **17**, 451–463.

Jokipii, L., Pohjola, S. and Jokipii, A.M.M. (1983) *Cryptosporidium*: a frequent finding in patients with gastrointestinal symptoms. *The Lancet*, **322**(8346), 358–361.

Jones, F., Kay, D., Stanwell-Smith, R. and Wyer, M. (1991) Results of the first pilot-scale controlled cohort epidemiological investigation into the possible health effects of bathing in seawater at Langland Bay, Swansea. *Journal of International Water and Environmental Management*, **5**, 91–97.

Kay, D., Jones, F., Wyer, M.D., Fleisher, J.M., Salmon, R.L., Godfree, A.F., Zelenauch-Jacquotte, A. and Shore, R. (1994) Predicting likelihood of gastroenteritis from sea bathing: results from randomised exposure. *The Lancet, 34***(8927),** 905–909.

Kay, D., Bartram, J., Prüss, A., Ashbolt, N., Wyer, M.D., Fleisher, J.M., Fewtrell, L., Rogers, A. and Rees, G. (2004) Derivation of numerical values for the World Health Organization guidelines for recreational waters. *Water Research*, **38**, 1296–1304.

Kosek, M., Alcantara, C., Lima, A.A.M. and Guerrant, R.L. (2001) Cryptosporidiosis: an update. *Lancet Infectious Diseases*, **1**(4), 262–269.

Kueh, C.S.W., Tam, T-Y. and Lee, T. (1995) Epidemiological study of swimming-associated illnesses relating to bathing-beach water quality. *Water Science and Technology*, **31**(5–6), 1–4.

Kuipers, E.J., Janssen, M.J.R. and de Boer, W.A. (2003) Good bugs and bad bugs: indications and therapies for *Helicobacter pylori* eradication. *Current Opinion in Pharmacology*, **3**(5), 480–485

Kuipers, E.J., Uyterlinde, A.M., Pena, A.S., Roosendaal, R., Pals, G., Nelis, G.F. Festen, H.P. and Meuwissen, S.G. (1995) Long term sequelae of *Helicobacter pylori* gastritis. *Lancet*, **345**(8964), 1525–1528.

Kuntz, T.B. and Kuntz, S.T. (1999) Enterohemorrhagic *E. coli* infection. *Primary Care Update for OB/GYNS*, **6**(6), 192–196

Kuroki, S., Saida, T., Nukina, M., Yoshioka, M. and Seino, J. (2001) Three patients with ophthalmoplegia associated with *Campylobacter jejuni*. *Pediatric Neurology*, **25**(1), 71–74.

Lane, S. and Lloyd, D. (2002) Current trends in research into the waterborne parasite *Giardia*. *Critical Reviews in Microbiology*, **28**(2), 123–114.

Larsson, A., Nilsson, B. and Eriksson, M. (1999) Thrombocytopenia and platelet microvesicle formation caused by *Legionella pneumophila* infection. *Thrombosis Research*, **96**(5,1), 391–397.

Lee, J.V., Dawson, S.R., Ward, S., Surman, S.B. and Neal, K.R. (1997) Bacteriophages are a better indicator of illness rates than bacteria amongst users of a white water course fed by a lowland river. *Water Science and Technology*, **35**(11–12), 165–170.

Levine, W. and Griffin, P. (1993) Vibrio infections on the Gulf Coast: results of first year regional surveillance. *Journal of Infectious Diseases*, **167**, 479–483.

Li, N., Bajoghli, A., Kubba, A. and Bhawan, J. (1999) Identification of mycobacterial DNA in cutaneous lesions of sarcoidosis. *Journal of Cutaneous Pathology*, **26**, 271–278.

Li, S., Culver, B. and Ren, J. (2003) Benefit and risk of exercise on myocardial function in diabetes. *Pharmacological Research*, **48**(2), 127–132.

Lightfoot, N.E. (1989) *A prospective study of swimming related illness at six freshwater beaches in Southern Ontario*. Unpublished PhD thesis. University of Toronto, Canada.

Lindsay, J.A. (1997) Chronic sequelae of food-borne disease. *Emerging Infectious Diseases*, **3**(4), 11 pp.

Loirat, C. (2001) Post-diarrhoea haemolytic-uraemic syndrome: clinical aspects. *Archives de Pédiatrie*, **8**(4), 776–784.

McBride, G.B., Bandaranayake, D.R., Salmond, C.E., Turner, S.J., Lewis, G., Till, D., Hatton, C. and Cooper, A.B. (1993) *Faecal indicator density and illness risk to swimmers in coastal waters: a preliminary study for New Zealand*. Proceedings of the Annual Conference of the New Zealand Water and Waste Association. Havelock North, New Zealand, 1–3 September 1993: 43–49.

McDonald, S.D. and Gruslin, A. (2001) A review of Campylobacter infection during pregnancy: a focus on *C. jejuni. Primary Care Update for OB/GYNS*, **8**(6), 253–257.

Martinez, A.J. (1993) Free-living amebas: infection of the central nervous system. *Mt Sinai Journal of Medicine*, **60**, 271–278.

Mead, P.S. and Griffin, P.M. (1998) *Escherichia coli* O157:H7. *Lancet*, **352**(9135), 1207–1212.

Medema, G.J., van Asperen, I.A., Klokman-Houweling, J.M., Nooitgedagt, A., van de Laar, M.J.W. and Havelaar, A.H. (1995) The relationship between health effects in triathletes and microbiological quality of freshwater. *Water Science and Technology*, **31**, 19–26.

Medema, G.J., van Asperen, I.A. and Havelaar, A.H. (1997) Assessment of the exposure of swimmers to microbiological contaminants in fresh waters. *Water Science and Technology*, **35**(11–12), 157–163.

Medical Research Council and Council for Scientific and Industrial Research (CSIR) (1995) *Pathogenic microorganisms/epidemiological – microbiological study.* Final report 1991–1995, South Africa.

Michel, M., Hayem, G., Rat, A.C., Meyer, O., Palazzo, E., Blétry, O. and Kahn, M.F. (1996) Complications infectieuses fatales chez deux patients atteints de maladie de Still de l'adulte. *La Revue de Médecine Interne*, **17**(5), 407–440.

Moore, B. (1959) Sewage contamination of coastal bathing waters in England and Wales: a bacteriological and epidemiological study. *Journal of Hygiene*, **57**, 435–472.

Mujeriego, R., Bravo, J.M. and Feliu, M.T. (1982) Recreation in coastal waters, public health implications. *Vièmes Journées Etud. Pollutions,* Cannes, CIESM, 585–594.

Nachamkin, I. (2002) Chronic effects of Campylobacter infection. *Microbes and Infection*, **4**(4), 399–403

National Centre for Social Research (1998) *Leisure day visits. Summary of the 1998 UK day visits survey.* Department for Culture, Media and Sport, London, United Kingdom.

New Jersey Department of Health (1989) *A study of the relationship between illness and ocean beach water quality.* Interim Summary Report, New Jersey Department of Health.

Nguyen, M.H., Stout, J.E. and Yu, V.L. (1991) Legionellosis. *Infectious Disease Clinics of North America,* **5**(3), 561–584.

NOAA (2004) 2005 National survey on recreation and the environment: a partnership planning for the eighth national recreational survey. Forest Service, NOAA, University of Georgia and University of Tennessee. Available online: www.srs.fs.usda.gov/trends/Nsre/NSRE200562303.pdf. Accessed 14th July 2005.

Parkin, R.T., Davies-Cole, J.O. and Balbus, J.M. (2000) A definition for chronic sequelae applied to campylobacter and Guillian-Barré syndrome (Gbs). *Annals of Epidemiology,* **10**(7), 473.

Philipp, R., Evan, E.J., Hughes, A.O., Grisdale, S.K., Enticott, R.G. and Jephcott, A.H. (1985) Health risks of snorkel swimming in untreated water. *International Journal of Epidemiology,* **14**(4), 624–627.

Pike, E.B. (1994) Health effects of sea bathing. *(WMI 9021) – Phase III: Final Report to the Department of the Environment (DoE).* Report No. DoE 3412/2. Water Research Centre plc, 1–38, Medmenham, United Kingdom.

Public Health Laboratory Service (1959) Sewage contamination of coastal bathing waters in England and Wales: a bacteriological and epidemiological study. *Journal of Hygiene,* **43**, 435–472.

Puleo Fadi, J.A., Matar, F.A., McKeown, P.P., Conant, P., Basta, L.L. (1995) Legionella pericarditis diagnosed by direct fluorescent antibody staining. *The Annals of Thoracic Surgery,* **60**(2), 444–446.

Prüss, A. (1998) Review of epidemiological studies on health effects from exposure to recreational water. *International Journal of Epidemiology,* **27**, 1–9.

Rahyaman, S.M., Chira, P. and Koff, R.S. (1994) Idiopathic autoimmune chronic hepatitis triggered by Hepatitis A. *American Journal of Gastroenterology,* **89**,106–108.

Reynolds, K. (2003) Collateral damage: The chronic sequelae of waterborne pathogens. *Water Conditioning and Purification Magazine,* **45**(8), 3pp. Available online http://www.wcp.net. Accessed 21 November 2003.

Rocha, H., Cruz, T., Brito, E. and Susin, M. (1976) Renal involvement in patients with hepatosplenic *Schistosomiasis mansoni. American Journal of Tropical Medicine and Hygiene.* **25**(1), 108–115.

Sasaki, D.M., Pang, L., Minette, H.P., Wakida, C.K., Fujimoto, W.J., Manea, S.J., Kunioka, R. and Middleton, C.R. (1993) Active surveillance and risk factors for leptospirosis in Hawaii. *American Journal of Tropical Medicine and Hygiene,* **48**(1), 35–43.

Seyfried, P.L., Tobin, R.S., Brown, N.E. and Ness, P.F. (1985) A prospective study of swimming related illness. I. Swimming associated health risk. *American Journal of Public Health,* **75**, 1068–1070.

Shpilberg, O., Shaked, Y., Maier, M.K. (1990) Long-term follow-up after leptospirosis. *Southern Medical Journal,* **83**(4), 405–407.

Shuval, H. (2003) Estimating the global burden of thalassogenic diseases: human infectious diseases caused by wastewater pollution of the marine environment. *Journal of Water and Health,* **1**(2), 53–64.

Simons, G.W., Hilscher, R., Ferguson, H.F. and Gage S. de M. (1922) Report of the Committee of Bathing Places. *American Journal of Public Health,* **12**(1), 121–123.

Singleton, P. and Sainsbury, D. (2001) *Dictionary of Microbiology and Molecular Biology,* 3rd edn, Wiley Europe.

Smythe, L., Dohnt, M., Symonds, M., Barnett, L., Moore, M., Brrookes, D. and Vallanjon, M. (2000) Review of leptospirosis notifications in Queensland and Australia: January 1998–June 1999. *Communicable Diseases Intelligence,* **24**(6), 153–157.

Soldatou, A. and Davies, E.G. (2003) Respiratory virus infections in the immunocompromised host. *Paediatric Respiratory Reviews,* **4**(3), 193–204.

Stevenson, A.H. (1953) Studies of bathing water quality and health. *American Journal of Public Health,* **43**, 529–538.

Tattevin, P. Dupeux, S and Hoff, J. (2003) Leptospirosis and the antiphospholipid syndrome. *The American Journal of Medicine,* **114**(2), 164.

Torre, D., Giola, M., Martegani, R., Zeroli, C., Fiori, G.P., Ferrario, G. and Bonetta, G. (1994) Aseptic meningitis caused by *Leptospira australis. European Journal of Clinical Microbiology and Infectious Diseases,* **13**, 496–497.

UNEP/WHO (1991) *Epidemiological studies related to environmental quality criteria for bathing waters, shellfish growing waters and edible marine waters (Activity D).* Final report on project on epidemiological study on bathers from selected beaches in Malaga, Spain (1988–1989), Athens, Greece. United Nations Environment Programme; MAP Technical Report Series No 53.

van Asperen, I.A., Medema, G., Borgdoff, M.W., Sprenger, M.J.W. and Havelaar, A.H. (1998) Risk of gastroenteritis among triathletes in relation to faecal pollution of freshwaters. *International Journal of Epidemiology,* **27,** 309–315.

Van Bohemen, Ch. G., Nabbe, A.J.J.M., Dinant, H.J., Grumet, F.C., Landheer, J.E. and Zanen, H.C. (1986) Lack of serologically defined arthritogenic *Shigella flexeri* cell envelope antigens in post-dysenteric arthritis. *Immunology Letters,* **13**(4), 197–201.

Van Dijk, P.A.H., Lacey, R.F. and Pike, E.B. (1996) *Health effects of sea-bathing – further analysis of data from UK beach surveys.* Final report to the Department of the Environment. Report No. 4126/3, Medmenham, UK, WRc plc.

Van de Vliet, P., Vanden Auweele, Y., Knapen, Y., Rzewnicki, R., Onghena, P. and Van Coppenolle, H. (2004) The effect of fitness training on clinically depressed patients: an intra-individual approach. *Psychology of Sport and Exercise,* **5**(2), 153–167.

Von Schirnding, Y.E., Kfir, R., Cabelli, V., Franklin, L., Joubert, G. (1992) Morbidity among bathers exposed to polluted seawater. A prospective epidemiological study. *South African Medical Journal,* **81,** 543–546.

Von Schirnding, Y.E.R., Straus, N., Robertson, P., Kifr, R., Fattal, B., Mahee, A., Frank, M and Cabelli, V.J. (1993) Bather morbidity from recreational exposure to sea water. *Water, Science and Technology,* **27**(3–4); 183–186.

Weiner, E.S. and Simpson, J. (1989) *The compact Oxford English dictionary.* 2nd edn, Oxford University Press, Oxford, UK.

WHO (1994) World Health Organization evaluation of carcinogenic risk to humans. Schistosome, liver flukes and *Helicobacter pylori. IARC Monographs,* **61,** 45–119.

WHO (2003a) *Guidelines for Safe Recreational Water Environments,* vol. 1, *Coastal and Freshwaters.* WHO, Geneva, Switzerland.

WHO (2003b) *Emerging issues in water and infectious diseases.* WHO, France.

WHO (2005) *Guidelines for Safe Recreational Water Environments,* vol. 2, *Swimming Pools, Spas and similar recreational-water Environments.* WHO, Geneva, Switzerland.

Willen, C., Stibrant, K., Sunnerhagen, S. and Grimby, G. (2001) Dynamic water exercise in individuals with late poliomyelitis. *Archives of Physical Medicine and Rehabilitation,* **82**(1), 66–72.

Wirguin, I., Briani, C., Suturkova-Milosevic, L., Fisher, T., Della-Latta, P., Chalif, P. and Latov, N. (1997) Induction of anti-GM1 ganglioside antibodies by *Campylobacter jejuni* lipopolysaccharides. *Journal of Neuroimmunology,* **78**(1–2), 138–142.

WTO (2001) Tourism 2020 vision volume 7: Global forecasts and profiles of market segments. World Tourism Organization, Madrid, Spain.

Yoder, J.S., Blackburn, B.G., Craun, G.F., Hill, V., Levy, D.A., Chen, N., Lee, S.H., Calderon, R.L. and Beach, M.J. (2004) Surveillance for waterborne-disease outbreaks associated with recreational water—United States, 2001–2002. US CDC, *MMWR, Surveillance Summaries,* October 22, 2004/53(SS08):1–22.

Yu, D.T. and Thompson, G.T. (1994) Clinical, epidemiological and pathogenic aspects of reactive arthritis. *Food Microbiology,* **11,** 97–108.

2

Hazard Identification and Factors Related to Infection and Disease

Assessment of the health impacts of recreational water quality is a useful tool in developing appropriate policies. Risk assessment approaches are increasingly being used as a scientific rationale for risk management. This chapter describes the various methods used for identification and quantification of hazards in recreational water risk assessment. It also looks at how different factors influence infection and disease.

2.1 HAZARD IDENTIFICATION

A hazard is a set of circumstances that could lead to harm. The existence of a wide range of hazards in the recreational water environment, such as physical hazards, water quality, contamination of beach sand, algae and their toxic products, chemical and physical agents and dangerous aquatic organisms, indicates a need for an understanding of their relative importance to health and the implications for control. Risk assessment models can assist in this process. The risk of harm occurring is defined as the probability that it will occur as a result of exposure to a defined quantum of hazard (Lacey and Pike 1989). The assessment of risk informs the development of policies for controlling and managing the risks to health and well-being in water recreation (WHO 2003).

2.1.1 Epidemiology

Identification of waterborne disease - both outbreaks and endemic disease - often relies on epidemiological investigations. Epidemiological studies are central to the assessment of risk by providing estimates of risk and data for risk assessment models. The aim of descriptive epidemiological investigations is to identify who was ill, the timing of the illness and the location. It is then possible to identify whether the same cases have been exposed to the same source. Confounding factors such as food consumption, age or gender should then be investigated and eliminated since they may bias the interpretation of the results of the study. These investigations will not confirm the route of transmission but may help to build a hypothesis about the cause of the illness which can then be further tested by an observational study.

The main types of epidemiological studies used to evaluate the health effects from bathing water pollution are cohort studies and randomised controlled trials. Cohort studies consider a group of people (the cohort), initially free of disease, who are classified into subgroups according to exposure to a potential cause of disease or outcome. Variables of interest are specified and measured and the whole cohort is followed up to see how the disease or outcome of interest differs between the groups with and without exposure. The data is collected at different points in time – prospective cohort studies are capable of estimating the associations of interest, but there may be variation in the composition of different exposure groups, there may be significant loss of follow-up subjects, and in some cases, the studies measure perception rather than the actual clinical incidence. In retrospective cohort studies the estimation of exposure can be significantly inaccurate because water quality can vary to a large degree both temporally and spatially (Kay and Dufour 2000).

In randomised controlled trials, subjects in a population are randomly allocated to groups – the control group and the treatment group, and the results of exposure are assessed by comparing the outcome in the two groups (see Box 2.1). Randomised controlled trials allow the accurate estimation of exposure to water, as well as water-quality assessments (Kay and Dufour 2000). However, these studies are costly and there are ethical problems relating to the need to ask volunteers to swim in contaminated waters.

A summary of major epidemiological studies undertaken in relation to illness associated with the use of recreational water and their findings are given in section 1.2. A description of randomized epidemiological studies is presented in Box 2.1.

Box 2.1 UK prospective randomised trial studies – assessing exposure

Randomised trials were conducted involving recruitment of healthy adult volunteers at seaside towns with adjacent beaches that had historically passed EU Imperative Standards (Jones *et al.* 1991; Kay *et al.* 1994). After initial interviews and medical checks, volunteers reported to the specified bathing location on the trial day where they were randomised into bather and non-bather groups.

Bathers entered the water at specified locations where intensive water quality monitoring was taking place. All bathers immersed their heads on three occasions. On exiting the water bathers were asked if they had swallowed water. The locations and times of exposure were known for each bather and, thus, a precise estimate of "exposure" (i.e. indicator bacterial concentration) could be assigned to each bather (Fleisher *et al.* 1993; Kay *et al.* 1994). A control group of non-bathers came to the beach and had a picnic of identical type to that provided for all volunteers. One week after exposure all volunteers returned for further interviews and medical examinations and later they completed a final postal questionnaire, three weeks after exposure.

Detailed water quality measurements were completed at defined "swim zones". Samples were collected synchronously at locations 20 m apart every 30 minutes and at three depths (i.e. surf zone, 1 m depth and at chest depth, 1.3–1.4 m). Five bacterial indicators were enumerated.

The analysis of the data centred on the links between water quality and gastroenteritis (see Fleisher *et al.* 1993; Kay *et al.* 1994). The data were analysed for relationships between water quality, as indexed by any of the five bacterial indicators measured at any of the three depths and gastroenteritis. Only faecal streptococci, measured at chest depth, provided a statistically significant relationship between water quality and the risk of gastroenteritis.

The limitations of UK randomised trial protocol include the fact that the studies were conducted in north European marine waters with a high tidal range where all waters commonly passed EU Imperative coliform criteria and the US EPA enterococci criteria (i.e., waters with relatively low faecal inputs). In addition, the results apply only to healthy adult volunteers, and may not be applicable directly to infants or chronically sick people or specialist user groups such as surfers.

2.1.2 Quantitative Microbial Risk Assessment

Quantitative Microbial Risk Assessment (QMRA) is used to estimate the probability of becoming infected by a specific pathogen after an exposure. QMRA uses densities of particular pathogens, assumed rates of ingestion, and appropriate dose-response models for the exposed population to estimate the level of risk (Haas *et al.* 1999). QMRA can be useful in determining the risk of infection from the use of recreational water. QMRA is theoretical but more predictive and sensitive and looks at the hazards, whereas epidemiological studies look at the disease using real data/observations. QMRA and epidemiological studies provide complimentary information and should be used together to provide better overall estimates of risk.

The process of QMRA produces a statistical estimate of adverse effects associated with exposure to particular hazards. The process consists of the following steps:

- Hazard identification (pathogen identification) – a qualitative determination of which pathogens threaten human health.
- Exposure assessment – a measurement or prediction of duration and intensity of exposure. Exposure is the likelihood of a human coming into contact with the hazard, which may be by ingestion, inhalation, contact etc.
- Dose-response assessment – an analysis of the probability of infection and/or disease which results from differing 'doses' of the pathogens (exposure duration and intensity).
- Risk characterisation – a combination of the above (Haas *et al.* 1999).

Two risk assessment studies investigating illness associated with recreational water have been carried out. Ashbolt *et al.* (1997) reported that the risks to bathers in Mamala Bay, Honolulu (Hawaii, USA), from enteric viruses were 10 to 100-fold greater than the risks from protozoa. However, bathers in Sydney, Australia had only slightly higher viral risks, assuming similar inactivation rates. Risks from bacterial pathogens and *Cryptosporidium* were significantly less in both studies. In both cases, the risks from entero- or adeno-virus infections were estimated to be between 10 and 50 people per 10,000 people exposed over seven days.

One of the main problems with risk assessment is that a number of assumptions need to be made with respect to exposures. Assumptions need to be validated through research under similar conditions to those being modelled. Slight changes in for example, pathogen concentration or die-off may lead to widely varying results.

In relation to using QMRA for recreational waters, data are currently lacking on behavioural patterns of recreational water users including the actual exposure level associated with inhalation, ingestion and skin contact with contaminated water and the corresponding level of illness that users experience. Although the frequency of illness or infections can be assessed through epidemiological studies in some cases, the factors that contribute to these adverse effects have not been well-quantified. However, this data is important since the degree of water contact directly influences the level of exposure to pathogens, toxic agents and other potential hazards and, therefore, the likelihood of contracting illness.

In 1951, Streeter attempted to develop a 'bather risk factor' (Streeter 1951). In order to do this he used the coliform-*Salmonella* ratio developed by Kehr and Butterfield (1943), the number of bathers exposed, the approximate volume of water ingested per day per bather and the average coliform density per ml of bathing water. More recent research has developed this approach further (see Box 2.1), and the relationship between the level of indicator species and the rates of illness has been used to derive the WHO *Guideline* values for microbial quality of recreational waters (WHO 2003). In marine environments, there is a direct correlation between concentrations of intestinal enterococci and both gastrointestinal illness and AFRI (WHO 2003).

2.2 FACTORS INFLUENCING HAZARD ENCOUNTER

2.2.1 Water contact

Water contact time is a prime factor influencing the amount of exposure to pathogens in water. The longer a person is in the water the more they can be exposed to pathogens in the water through ingestion, inhalation or penetration of the skin (e.g., schistosomiasis). The US EPA estimates that 100 ml of water enters the mouth and nasopharynx during a typical swimming episode (US EPA 1999). Review of the literature did not reveal any published estimates of the quantities of water ingested during recreational water activities other than swimming or provide estimates of average immersion times.

Some activities are likely to pose greater risk of water ingestion than others. The British Sub Aqua Club for example estimates that in winter the average length of a scuba dive is between 20 minutes and 30 minutes but in summer it can be more than one hour (Alistair Reynolds, British Sub Aqua Club Technical Manager, personal communication, 2001). The average volume of water consumed during a typical dive is not known. A study of scuba divers from New York City's police and fire departments indicated an association between scuba diving and gastrointestinal illness (Anonymous 1983). The divers reported ingesting small quantities of water while swimming at the surface and while using mouthpieces that had dangled in the water before use. Stool samples revealed 12 cases of gastrointestinal parasites – five of *Entamoeba histolytica* and seven of *Giardia lamblia*. One bacterial culture was positive for *Campylobacter*. Twenty-three non-diving fire-fighters had stools examined for parasites; none had *G. lamblia* or *E. histolytica*.

In recent years the popularity of activities which involve contact with water has grown and the increasing availability of the wet suit has altered the public use of recreational water especially in temperate regions with colder water. Prolonged periods of immersion are now becoming normal and activity occurs throughout the year and not just during the bathing seasons. Many gastrointestinal infections occur on a seasonal basis and therefore users will be exposed to different types of pathogens in the water. The density of users (bather-loads) at smaller recreational water bodies, especially where there is limited water turnover, may be a significant factor in the user-to-user transmission of disease. The personal hygiene of recreational water users while in the water (which may also significantly alter the quality of the water) is also a concern. A number of *Cryptosporidium* outbreaks in pools are thought to have been caused by swimmers who have had 'faecal accidents' (Lee *et al.* 2002; WHO, 2005). In addition, certain activities that increase the likelihood of ingestion of water, e.g. surfing, may lead to higher levels of risk (WHO, 2003).

Skin abrasions or cuts may contribute to recreational water-associated infections. Many environmental bacteria such as species of *Pseudomonas*, *Aeromonas*, and halophilic vibrios are opportunistic pathogens that may cause wound infections. In some cases, these infections can be life-threatening, e.g. *Vibrio vulnificus* (Chang *et al.* 1997).

2.2.2 Recreational water types

In discussing the health implications of using recreational waters, marine, freshwaters and enclosed pools, including hot tubs and spas, should be considered, as the different characteristics of the water bodies influence the hazards that may be encountered. Freshwater bathing sites may be enclosed bodies of water and fairly static, such as lakes, or running waters such as rivers. Both have features that require special consideration to protect water users. The concentration of pathogens is largely determined by faecal pollution from both point and non-point sources, although in some tropical/subtropical waters some species (e.g., *Vibrio* spp.) may be able to grow and support self sufficient populations (WHO 2004). Major point sources of pollution include sewage effluents, combined sewer overflows, industrial effluents and concentrated animal feeding operations. Non-point sources of pollution relate to agricultural activity and poorly functioning sanitation systems within the watershed, and are influenced by the type and density of livestock and other animals that might be present. Pathogen inputs may also exhibit seasonal variations, for example *Cryptosporidium* concentrations may be highest during the periods of calving or lambing (Reilly and Browning 2004). Urban surfaces also contribute significantly to the pollution load by discharging surface contaminants including animal faeces into sewers and storm drains.

Faecal material is transported from the watershed surface into rivers, lakes and streams, as well as directly via sewage discharge, and subsequently to the coastal environment. The transport of microbial and other contamination is controlled by the flow of water, and changes in flow are determined by rainfall and by the hydrogeological characteristics of the basin which have a significant impact on the concentration of microbes transported. In riverbed sediments the survival times of some pathogens are significantly increased (WHO 2003) and they may be resuspended when the river flow increases (Ferley *et al.* 1989; Environment Agency of England and Wales 2000). The survival of pathogenic microorganisms in water is impacted by temperature, light intensity, salinity and water quality (Johnson *et al.* 1997). In general, most excreta-related pathogens survive for longer periods of time in colder waters (Feachem *et al.* 1983).

Swimming pools and spas present special conditions that may result in different exposures or favour the growth/survival of specific pathogens. Leisure pools and hot tubs may be subject to higher bather loads than naturally occurring recreational waters, increasing the likelihood of water pollution from the bathers themselves and subsequent person-to-person transmission of disease. Chlorination of pool water will generally significantly reduce the concentrations of faecally-related bacteria (e.g., *E. coli*) but will have little or no impact on some protozoan parasites such as *Cryptosporidium*. Thus, waterborne outbreaks associated with exposure to chlorinated waters are much more likely to be caused by *Cryptosporidium* than the faecally-derived bacteria (Yoder *et al.* 2002).

Non-faecal shedding in the water is a source of potential non-enteric pathogenic organisms. Infected users can directly contaminate the pool, hot tub or spa water and the surfaces surrounding the pool with pathogens such as viruses and fungi, which can lead to skin infections such as verrucas.

Higher water temperatures favour the growth of some organisms such as *Legionella*. Pools without water treatment may be associated with higher risk of transmission among users.

Certain free-living bacteria and amoebas can grow in pool, hot tub and spa waters and in the heating, ventilation and air conditioning, causing a variety of respiratory, dermal or central nervous system infections or diseases (WHO 2003). Growth of certain free-living bacteria, such as *Vibrio vulnificus*, is favoured in warm marine water temperatures. Seasonal growth may occur – *V. vulnificus* has been shown to enter a viable but non-culturable state, a survival response to low-temperature stress (Wolf and Oliver 1992).

In both coastal and freshwaters the point sources of pollution that cause most health concern are those due to domestic sewage discharges, riverine discharges and contamination from bathers. The relative risks to human health from these sources depend on a number of factors. For example, sewage being discharged into an estuary with small tidal interchanges may have a different effect to that of the same quantity of sewage being discharged into an estuary with large tidal interchanges. Areas with direct discharge of crude, untreated or inadequately treated sewage are likely to present a higher risk to public health. The content of raw or inadequately treated sewage reflects the health status of the population it is derived from. Higher concentrations of pathogens will be present in areas where there is more disease or during disease outbreaks. This presents a special risk for people coming from low-pathogen circulation environments to high-pathogen circulation environments. Visitors may be at a greater risk than local populations. Information on local circumstances should be taken into account when setting guidelines to protect public health and these may vary locally or regionally. Further information on guideline setting can be found in the WHO *Guidelines for Safe Recreational Water Environments* (WHO 2003; WHO 2005).

2.3 FACTORS RELATED TO INFECTION AND DISEASE

2.3.1 Status of host

Of particular importance to the discussion of health risks associated with recreational use of water is the status of the immune system of a water user which will determine their susceptibility to infection and the severity of resulting illness. Tzipori (1988) speculated that the lower prevalence of cryptosporidiosis in older children and adults is due to immunity acquired from prior exposure. The immune status of the host seems to be the major determinant of whether the infection is self-limiting or persistent. Dysfunction of the T-lymphocytes and hypogammoglobulinaemia can both lead to persistent cryptosporidiosis (Tzipori 1988).

Research has shown that persistent over-training by athletes as well as a single bout of heavy exercise can increase susceptibility to upper respiratory and other viral infections, although resistance to bacterial infections appears to be unaltered. Heavy exercise, which in the context of this review may refer to competitive swimming training for example, appears to have a depressant effect on the T cell/interleukin/NK cell system which may remain for a week or more. In contrast, moderate training seems to enhance the immune status (Radak *et al.* 1999). It may be possible to infer from this research that competitive swimmers could be more at risk from contracting upper respiratory and viral infections than non-competitive recreational water users.

On the other hand, certain segments of the population are especially vulnerable to acute illness (morbidity) and can exhibit high death rates. These segments include those whose immune systems are compromised by illnesses such as cancer, AIDS or the drugs used to treat these and other conditions, the elderly, young children and pregnant women. Table 2.1 shows the estimated percentage of the population in the United States that are at risk of reduced immune function due to certain characteristics or disease. Categories are not mutually exclusive.

Table 2.1 Selected subpopulations in the United States at risk of reduced immune function

Subpopulation	Estimated percentage of population
Pregnant women (Ventura *et al.* 1999)	2.4
Infants and children (<10 years) (US Census Bureau 2000)	14.1
Elderly (65+ years) (US Census Bureau 2000)	12.6
Health status	
Diabetes (diagnosed and estimated undiagnosed cases) (CDC 2003)	6.3
Liver impairments (US EPA 1998)	0.2
Cardiovascular disease (http://www.nhlbi.nih.gov/)	21.7
AIDS (CDC 1999)	0.2

Table 2.2 Prevalence of 'at risk' persons in the domestic setting in selected European countries (Adapted from Exner and Kistemann 2003).

	The United Kingdom	Germany	The Netherlands
Total population	60 million	82 million	16 million
Elderly (65+ years)	9 million	13 million	2 million
Under one year old	600,000	800,000	100,000
Living with cancer	1 million	Data not available	160,000
Discharged from hospital within previous two weeks	200,000	Data not available	100,000
Hospital outpatients at home	Data not available	1,270,000	Data not available
AIDS cases	15,000	Data not available	91
Total 'at risk' persons	>1 in 6	>1 in 5.6	>1 in 6.3

Infectious diseases are a major problem in the elderly because the immune system declines with age, antibiotic treatment is less effective because a decrease in physiological function and malnutrition is more common (Meyers 1989). Nursing home studies have shown dramatic increases in diarrhoeal deaths in individuals over age 55, with mortality rates as high as 1 in 100, or 10 to 100 times greater than in the general population (Gerba *et al.* 1996). Skirrow (1994) and Allos and Blaser (1995) report that 0.6% of adults over the age of 65 develop bacteraemia following infection with *Campylobacter jejuni*, compared with between 0.15% and 0.4% in the general population. Other subpopulations at increased risk from infection are women during pregnancy, neonates and young children. Gust and Purcell (1987) and Craske (1992) report case-fatality ratios ranging from 1% to 2% in tourists from within the United States contracting HEV compared with case-fatality ratios of between 10% and 20% and even as high as 40% in pregnant women.

Infection during pregnancy may also result in the transmission of infection from the mother to the child *in utero*, during birth, or immediately afterwards (Gerba *et al.* 1996). Coxsackie- and echo-viruses appear to be transmitted in this way. An average case-fatality of 3.4% was observed in 16 documented outbreaks of echovirus in newborn nurseries (Modlin and Kinney 1987). In two outbreaks of coxsackie B virus in nurseries, the infant mortality rate from myocarditis ranged from 50% to 60% (Modlin and Kinney 1987).

The impact of AIDS has been shown to increase the number of diarrhoeal deaths in the age group 25 to 54 years (Lew *et al.* 1991). Enteric bacterial infections are more severe in people infected with AIDS/HIV. Although people with AIDS/HIV may not have more severe illness with *Giardia*, they have been shown to exhibit impaired immune response to the parasite (Mandell *et al.* 1990). AIDS increases the incidence of *Campylobacter*-associated enteritis to 519 per 100,000, at least 39 times higher than that of the general population (Alketruse *et al.* 1999). Baine *et al.* (1982) and Gorbach *et al.* (1992) have demonstrated that people with AIDS/HIV with infections from *Salmonella* spp., *Shigella* spp., and *Campylobacter* spp. often develop bacteraemia.

Cryptosporidiosis has been a serious problem for people with AIDS/HIV (Fahey 2003). It has since been on the rise as a cause of chronic diarrhoea in the immunosuppressed population (Guerrant 1997). Symptoms may persist for many months with severe and protracted diarrhoea, resulting in weight loss and mortality. Mortality rates of 50% have been reported for this organism (Clifford *et al.* 1990).

People with cancer may undergo intensive treatment which often supresses the immune system. Hierholzer (1992) has shown that in immunosuppressed patients due to cancer treatment, the fatality rate for patients infected with certain adenovirus strains can be as high as 53%.

In contrast to many of the other enteric viruses, neither Norovirus nor HAV appear to be associated with a greater severity or chronic illness in the immunocompromised (Rubin and Young 1988).

2.3.2 Process of infection

The hazards that are encountered in recreational water environments vary from site-to-site and by the type of activity. Most available information relates to health outcomes arising from exposure through swimming and ingestion of contaminated water. Recreational waters generally contain a mixture of pathogenic and non-pathogenic microbes. These microbes may be derived from sewage effluents, the population using the water, livestock or other animals, industrial processes, farming activities (e.g., use of animal manures as fertilisers), as well as indigenous pathogenic micro-organisms. Bathers may succumb to infection when an organism colonises a suitable growth site in the body. These sites are typically the alimentary canal, eyes, ears, nasal cavity and upper respiratory tract and may also include opportunistic colonisation of wound infections. Depending on their route of transmission, waterborne pathogens can be classified into those that are transmitted via ingestion and those that are transmitted via inhalation or contact. Transmission pathways for some pathogens are given in Table 2.3.

Table 2.3 Transmission pathways for a selection of waterborne pathogens (Exner and Kistemann 2002; Chang *et al.* 1997).

Ingestion	Inhalation	Contact	Wound Infections
V. cholera	*Legionella* spp.	*P. aeruginosa*	*Aeromonas* spp.
Salmonella spp.	*Mycobacteria* spp.	*Aeromonas* spp.	*Pseudomonas* spp.
E. coli		*Mycobacteria* spp.	*Vibrio vulnificus*
Shigella spp.		*Acanthamoeba* spp.	*Vibrio parahaemolyticus*
Campylobacter spp.		*Naegleria* spp.	
Helicobacter spp.		Schistosoma.	
Enteroviruses			
Noroviruses			
Hepatoviruses			
Rotaviruses			

The infectivity of a pathogen depends upon the form it is in when encountered, the conditions of exposure and the host's susceptibility and immune status. The dose required to initiate an infection may be very few viable units, especially where viral and parasitic protozoan pathogens are concerned (Fewtrell *et al.* 1993; Okhuysen and Chappell 2002), e.g. HAV or *Cryptosporidium*. In reality, recreational water users rarely encounter a single pathogen, and the effects of multiple and simultaneous exposures to pathogens are poorly understood (Esrey *et al.* 1985).

Pathogens have various properties for increasing their ability to cause disease (including their ability to survive and proliferate in the environment), of particular relevance are those that facilitate attachment, invasion and replication in the host (Archer and Young 1988; Bunning 1994; Bunning *et al.* 1997). In addition, a pathogen's ability to evade the host's immune system plays a major role in determining the ability of the pathogen to cause disease. With enteric viruses, age plays an important role in the probability of developing clinical illness. For example, for HAV the percentage of individuals with clinically observed illness is low for children but increases greatly with age. In contrast, the frequency of clinical symptoms for group A rotavirus infections is greatest in childhood and lowest in adulthood (Bosch 1998).

The range of host response to infection depends upon the agent and the host and varies from subclinical infection (i.e. infection in which symptoms are not apparent) to primary disease response and, in some individuals, sequelae (refer to section 1.3 for further discussion).

Modlin, J.F. and Kinney, J.S. (1987) Prenatal enterovirus infections. *Advances in Pediatric Infectious Disease*, **2**(8), 918–926.

Okhuysen, P.C. and Chappell, C.L. (2002) *Cryptosporidium* virulence determinants – are we there yet? *International Journal for Parasitology*, **32**(5), 517–525.

Radak, Z., Kaneko, T., Tahara, S., Nakamoto, H., Ohno, H., Sasvari, M., Nyakas, C. and Goto, S. (1999) The effect of exercise training on oxidative damage of lipids, proteins, and DNA in rat skeletal muscle: evidence for beneficial outcomes. *Free Radical Biology and Medicine,* **27**(1–2), 67–74.

Reilly, W.J. and Browning, L.M. (2004) Zoonoses in Scotland - food, water, or contact? (Chapter 11). In: Cotruvo, J.A., Dufour, A., Rees, G., Bartram, J., Carr, R., Cliver, D.O., Craun, G.F., Fayer, R., and Gannon, V.P.J. (eds.) *Waterborne Zoonoses: Identification, Causes and Control.* Published on behalf of the World Health Organization by IWA Publishing, London.

Rubin, R.H. and Young, L.S. (1988) *Clinical approach to infection in the compromised host.* Second Edition. Plenum Press, New York.

Skirrow, M.B. (1994) Diseases due to Campylobacter, Helicobacter and related bacteria. *Journal of Comparative Pathology,* **111**, 113–149.

Streeter, H.W. (1951) *Bacterial-quality objectives for the Ohio River.* Ohio River Valley Water Sanitation Commission, Cincinnati, United States.

Tzipori, S. (1988) Cryptosporidiosis in perspective. *Advances in Parasitology,* **27**, 63–129.

US Census Bureau. (2000) *Resident population estimates of the United States by age and sex. April 1, 1990 to July 1, 1999 with short-term projection to July 1, 2000.* Population Estimates Program, Population Division, US Census Bureau, Washington, DC, USA.

US Environmental Protection Agency (US EPA) (1998) *Demographic distribution of sensitive population groups. Office of Science and Technology/ Office of Water, US Environmental Protection Agency.* Prepared by SRA Technologies, Inc. (ed. R. O'Day, J. Rench, R. Oen, and A. Castro), Fall Church, USA.

US Environmental Protection Agency (US EPA). (1999) *Action Plan for Beaches and Recreational Waters.* Available online: http://www.epa.gove/ORD/publications.

Ventura, S.J., Mosher, W.D., Curtin, S.C., Abma, J.C. and Henshaw, S. (1999) Highlights of trends in pregnancies and pregnancy rates by outcome: Estimates for the United States, 1976–1996. *National vital statistics reports,* **47**(29). National Centre for Health Statistics, Hyattsville, USA.

Wolf, P.W. and Oliver, J.D. (1992) Temperature effects on the viable but nonculturable state of *Vibrio vulnificus. FEMS Microbiology Letters,* **101**, 33–39.

WHO (2000) *The increasing incidence of human campylobacteriosis. Report and proceedings of a WHO consultation of experts.* WHO/CDS/CSR/APH/2000.4. World Health Organization, Copenhagen, Denmark.

WHO (2001) *Waterborne disease surveillance: Goals and strategies. Report on a meeting of a working group.* Budapest, Hungary, November 2001. World Health Organization, Copenhagen, Denmark.

WHO (2003) *Guidelines for Safe Recreational Water Environments, vol. 1, Coastal and Freshwaters.* World Health Organization, Geneva, Switzerland.

WHO (2004) Guidelines for Safe Drinking Water, 3rd Edition, WHO, Geneva.

WHO (2005) *Guidelines for Safe Recreational Water Environments,* vol. 2, *Swimming Pools, Spas and similar recreational-water Environments.* WHO, Geneva, Switzerland.

3

Credibility of Association and Severity Criteria Index

This chapter presents a modified framework for assessing the credibility of association of illness with recreational water exposures and presents information on waterborne disease surveillance systems. Evidence for severity is outlined and an index of severity is described to help public health professionals better prioritize and manage diseases with potentially severe outcomes related to recreational water exposures.

3.1 SOURCES OF AVAILABLE EVIDENCE

Evidence for this review is taken from two main sources: published scientific literature (case reports and epidemiological studies) accessed through databases such as MEDLINE; and available data reported to national surveillance centres. The majority of cases of illnesses associated with recreational waters are reported from the United States and the United Kingdom (the latter since 1992) due to the nature of surveillance systems in place in those countries. Where possible, peer-reviewed cases or government-reported data from other countries have been included.

Data for this review has also been obtained from a database of illnesses reported by the general public developed and maintained by Surfers Against Sewage (a United Kingdom-based pressure group). There are currently over 800 cases reported on the database, which exhibit a broad range of symptoms from mild to severe. It should be stressed that this is not an official surveillance system, but a self-reporting system.

3.1.1 Limitations of the evidence

As Table 1.1 illustrates a number of targeted epidemiological studies on infectious diseases associated with recreational water contact have been conducted. These studies demonstrate an association between recreational water contact and infectious disease transmission. However, infections and illnesses due to recreational water contact are generally mild and so difficult to detect through routine surveillance systems. Even where illness is more severe, it may still be difficult to attribute to recreational water exposure. Many of the pathogens that can be transmitted through recreational water contact can also be transmitted through other waterborne routes, through food and by person-to-person contact. As discussed in section 2.1.1. epidemiological studies are often difficult and expensive to perform (Teunis and Havelaar 2002). Waterborne outbreaks are often associated with contamination events, but these occur at unpredictable intervals and early warning seldom occurs, so that reliable exposure data immediately before and during outbreaks are infrequently available.

3.2 SURVEILLANCE

The likelihood of an outbreak coming to the attention of health authorities varies considerably depending on the department's interest in waterborne diseases and its budgetary, investigative and laboratory resources. Additionally, a few outbreaks involving very large numbers of people may alter the relative proportion of cases attributed to specific etiologic agents.

Waterborne disease surveillance requires the detection of increased illness in a population and evidence to show that water was the route of transmission. Tillett *et al.* (1998) describes a number of problems with identifying waterborne disease. One of these relates to detecting clinical cases; unless patients seek medical advice, cases will go undetected. Where medical assistance is sought and faecal specimens are taken, an increase in the number of referrals may be noted by the diagnostic laboratories. Where samples give a positive microbiological result there is the opportunity to detect increases in cases of that diagnosis by the laboratory or the public health department where laboratory data are collated.

Monitoring disease patterns by laboratory reports is useful but is susceptible to biases such as under-reporting, under-detection and changes in laboratory methods. These biases will particularly affect geographical comparisons. Many waterborne pathogens are also spread by routes of transmission other than water and therefore observed increases may not be waterborne. Where no causative organism is found, the disease will not be detected through the laboratory reporting method.

In some cases increased surveillance of illness results from the reporting of a water contamination incident. However, the quality of the water is usually investigated only after a cluster of clinical cases are discovered and water is suspected of being a possible route of transmission. By the time disease is detected and investigated the water quality may have changed, the flow of natural water or the changeover in artificial pools may leave no evidence as to the water quality at the relevant time. In addition, routine monitoring of recreational sites measures indicator organisms and not pathogens - and is not conducted in real time. Furthermore, the microbiological quality of water will change during storage, making retrospective analysis of contaminated samples very unreliable.

In some parts of the United States, a comprehensive programme of surveillance has been established (see box 3.1). In Milwaukee, Wisconsin for example, as a result of the *Cryptosporidium* outbreak in 1993, a community action and response plan was developed in the event of a waterborne disease emergency. Specific 'trigger' events have been identified (such as breach of the total coliform rule, exceedence of surface water standards, breakdown of water filtration equipment, unusual number of customer complaints about water quality, pathogens found in the treated water, increased reports of diarrhoeal illness or laboratory-confirmed cases reported to local health departments); levels of response to the trigger events (such as levels of health risk suspected and recommended action); and advice about who should be notified in the event of an emergency.

Proctor *et al.* (1998) compared the advantages and disadvantages of the surveillance data available during the outbreak of *Cryptosporidium* in Milwaukee, Wisconsin, the United States. The authors highlighted the weaknesses in all proposed waterborne surveillance systems. For example, treated water can meet all US water quality standards and yet still contain sufficient pathogens to cause a community-wide disease outbreak. Increased prevalence of diarrhoeal disease (and other diseases) in some populations need to be interpreted with caution because a variety of (gastrointestinal) problems can exist in some vulnerable sections of the population such as the elderly or immunocompromised. The epidemiological use of drug prescriptions as markers of disease have been used in some countries (see for example Maggini *et al.* 1991 and Miller *et al.* 1997).

Box 3.1 CDC Waterborne Disease Surveillance System

In the United States, the CDC maintains a database of waterborne disease outbreaks. The database is compiled based upon responses to a voluntary and confidential survey form that is completed by some state and local public health officials. CDC request reports from state and territorial epidemiologists or from people designated as the Waterborne Disease Outbreak (WBDO) surveillance co-ordinators. CDC and US EPA believe that many disease outbreaks are not reported to the CDC and, therefore, are under-represented by the survey. Craun *et al.* (1996) reports that outbreaks are not recognised unless approximately 1% or more of the exposed population becomes ill.

The WBDO surveillance system records outbreaks rather than individual cases of a particular disease. An outbreak is constituted as two or more persons having experienced a similar illness after exposure to water used for recreational purposes (Levy *et al.* 1998). This stipulation is waived for single cases of laboratory confirmed primary amebic meningoencephalitis (PAM). Secondly, epidemiological evidence must implicate water as the probable source of the illness.

If primary and secondary cases are distinguished on the outbreak form, only primary case counts are included in the total number of cases. If both actual and estimated case counts are included on the report form, the estimated count is used if the study population was sampled randomly or was calculated using the attack rate.

The surveillance system classifies WBDOs according to the strength of the evidence implicating water as the source of the outbreak. The classification numbers are based on the epidemiological and water quality data provided on the outbreak form. Epidemiological data is weighted more heavily than water quality data. The cases with water quality data but no epidemiological data are not included in the CDC reports. Recreational waters include swimming pools, hot tubs, spas, water parks, and naturally occurring fresh and marine surface waters according to CDC. It does not encompass wound infections resulting from waterborne organisms such as *Aeromonas* spp.

No single set of recommended surveillances will be applicable to all communities, a combination of surveillance options should be developed locally. Proctor *et al.* (1998) conclude that the most effective waterborne illness surveillance systems are those which can easily be linked to laboratory data, are flexible in adding new variables, and which show low baseline data variability. In addition to the importance of having baseline data for the recognition of unusual occurrences, a community-wide plan for critically and systematically evaluating the data is as important.

Illnesses reported by surveillance systems probably represent significant underestimates of illness associated with waterborne disease agents (WHO 2001). The reasons may vary but will include under-reporting of sporadic cases.

Outbreaks or sporadic illness occurring due to opportunistic pathogens that may be widespread in recreational waters may not be detectable by surveillance systems but may cause illness with insidious onset and long incubation periods in persons who are immunocompromised. Their limitations notwithstanding, surveillance data do yield information on the types of water systems and their deficiencies, their water quality, and the disease agents associated with outbreaks. These data may be used to evaluate the relative degrees of risk associated with different types of water, problems in current technologies and operating conditions, and the adequacy of current regulations (Craun *et al.* 2002).

3.3 CREDIBILITY OF ASSOCIATION WITH RECREATIONAL WATER

In this review a 'weight of evidence' approach has been developed to establish the credibility of association of an illness with recreational water exposure. The approach is based on a framework developed by the Communicable Disease Surveillance Centre (CDSC) in the United Kingdom used to assess whether a disease was associated with a water-related exposure route (Anonymous 1996). The approach takes into account epidemiology, microbiology and water quality information. Outbreaks are therefore categorised as being associated with water 'strongly', 'probably' or 'possibly', identified as below. Anecdotal information is not accepted by the CDSC.

Credibility of association with recreational water:

Strongly associated
- Evidence exists from at least one well-described outbreak where a case controlled/cohort study found a significant association with recreational water contact.
  Or
- Descriptive epidemiology suggests a link to recreational water **and** evidence exists to show that the pathogen was isolated from recreational waters.
  Or
- A well-designed prospective epidemiological study of sporadic illness found a significant association with recreational water contact.

Probably associated:
- Evidence from the literature suggests a biologically plausible association between recreational use of water and the disease symptoms but no pathogen was isolated from the water at the time of investigation.

Possibly associated:
- The pathogen has been isolated from a recreational water body but there is no supporting evidence.
  Or
- Where other evidence suggests that a water route is plausible.

3.4 EVIDENCE FOR SEVERITY

Fleisher *et al.* (1998) undertook the first epidemiological study to assess and report the severity of illnesses associated with bathing in recreational waters contaminated with domestic sewage. This was based on the results of randomized intervention trials at four bathing locations in the United Kingdom of acceptable quality according to EU and US EPA criteria. Severity was based on three outcome measures – duration of illness, whether or not the individual sought medical attention (Table 3.1), and the number of days of normal activity lost due to the particular ailment (Table 3.2). The authors concluded that gastroenteritis, AFRI, eye and ear ailments cannot be considered as 'minor' illnesses.

Table 3.1 Duration of illness and percentage of bathers seeking medical attention (Adapted from Fleisher *et al.* 1998).

Ailment	Mean duration of illness (days)	Percentage of bathers seeking medical attention
Gastroenteritis	4	12.0
AFRI	6	22.2
Ear ailments	8	20.9
Eye ailments	4	4.2

Table 3.2 Mean number of days of normal activity lost due to bathing-related illness (Adapted from Fleisher *et al.* 1998).

Ailment	Percentage of bathers losing at least one day	Percentage of bathers losing two days	Percentage of bathers losing three days
Gastroenteritis	14.7	4	1.4
AFRI	7.4	14.8	3.7
Ear ailments	2.3	2.3	2.3
Eye ailments	4.2	8.3	0

3.4.1 Severity Index

For the purposes of this review a simplified index of severity has been created and applied wherever possible to the illnesses considered, taking into account possible sequelae. The index is limited by the availability of data and does not take into account the probability of infection following exposure. The index is designed to help public health professionals prioritize recreational water management decisions to reduce the potential for severe disease outcomes.

The outcome measures used to ascertain the relative severity are case-fatality rate, average duration of illness, median percentage of cases requiring hospitalisation, the frequency of development of sequelae and the severity of sequelae. For each component of the severity index a score is given as shown in Table 3.3. Data has been used from published reports (as indicated in Tables 3.4–3.6) to produce the final scores in Tables 3.7–3.9. In some cases data is not available and this has been indicated. Case-fatality from *H. pylori* is unknown for example – median figure given as estimate.

It should be emphasised that these data are only valid for certain regions of the world since not all pathogens are found worldwide, and some data are estimates. This gives an indication of the severity and does not take into account prevalence. For example, for most people infected *by N. fowleri* the infection is extremely severe. However, the prevalence is low. Ameobic encephalitis may result in very severe outcomes, even death, but the prevalence of the illness may be very low. The determination of the severity of the illness, together with the prevalence of the illness in a given location caused by the pathogens described can be useful to allow water quality managers to prioritise their management needs. In this context managers must apply a risk-benefit approach to management (see Table 3.10 for examples of different management actions that might be possible for different types of pathogens).

It should be borne in mind that the spectrum and severity of disease in immunocompromised individuals is greater than in immunocompetent people. For example, immunocompromised individuals with cryptosporidiosis illustrate this since the most severe disease is seen in individuals with defects in the T-cell response. People with AIDS suffer from more severe and prolonged gastrointestinal disease that can be fatal; in addition, internal organs other than the gastrointestinal tract may be affected (Hunter and Nichols 2002).

The severity of an illness depends on a variety of factors, as discussed in section 1.3. When an individual is exposed to a pathogen, a range of health outcomes is possible. The person may be infected without noticing any symptoms or may become ill with mild symptoms or severe symptoms. This effect is true for both healthy and susceptible individuals. The precise health outcome for a particular person exposed and a particular pathogen is often not predictable. Some pathogens have very specific survival conditions, others are very robust. As Tables 3.7–3.9 show the severity of the illness can be increased dramatically in immunocompromised persons.

Table 3.3 Computation of severity score.

Case-fatality		Acute illness						Sequelae	
Rate (%)	Score	Median % requiring hospitalisation	Score	Duration	Score	Frequency of development (% of cases)	Score	Severity	Score
<1%	1	<1%	1	<48 hours	1	<1	1	No disability or interference with daily life	0
1–3.9%	2	1–5%	2	2–4 days	2	1–5	2	Interferes with daily life	1
4–5.9%	3	5–10%	3	4–8 days	3	5–10	3	Prolonged hospitalisation	2
6–7.9%	4	10–20%	4	8–16 days	4	10–20	4	May result in death	3
8–9.9%	5	>20%	5	>16 days	5	>20	5		
>10%	6								

Table 3.4 Summary of data used to compile severity scores (bacteria).

Pathogenic agent	Case-fatality rate (%) in immunocompetent patients	Case-fatality rate (%) in immunocompromised / sensitive groups	Severity of acute illness (Median % requiring hospitalisation)	Duration of acute illness	Frequency of sequelae (% of cases developing sequelae)	Severity of sequelae	Availability of treatment/ vaccine
Campylobacter spp.	0.4% (4 deaths per 1000 infections) (WHO 2000)	AIDS patients particularly susceptible	13% (New Zealand Food Safety Authority 2001)	1 day to 3 weeks (Allos and Blaser 1995)	0.1% (1 in 1000) develop Guillain-Barré syndrome (United States; Buzby et al. 1997)	Interferes with daily life	Antibiotic treatment available.
Shiga toxin-producing *E. coli*	0.8% (New Zealand Food Safety Authority 2001)	No data available but children, the elderly and immunocompromised are most at risk from developing severe complications.	29.5% (New Zealand Food Safety Authority 2001)	5 days or less	2–8% will develop HUS (Lansbury and Ludlam 1997)	Prolonged hospitalisation, death	Antibiotic treatment available.
Helicobacter pylori	High if progresses to gastric cancer; high (6–10%) if haemorrhage from peptic ulcer occurs otherwise unknown, likely to be low.	No data found	0.04% (United States; CDC 2003a)	Gastritis lasts several days to weeks	15% (WHO 2003)	Can result in cancer – may result in death, ulcers also debilitating	Antibiotic treatment available.
Legionella spp. causing Legionnaires disease	15% (Barbaro 2002) 15–20% (Mandell et al. 1990)	80% in immunosuppressed patients (Mandell et al. 1990).	2–15% (Muder et al. 1989)	6–7 days	2–16% (Bohte et al. 1995)	Prolonged hospitalisation	Antibiotic treatment available.

Pathogenic agent	Case-fatality rate (%) in immunocompetent patients	Case-fatality rate (%) in immunocompromised / sensitive groups	Severity of acute illness (Median % requiring hospitalisation)	Duration of acute illness	Frequency of sequelae (% of cases developing sequelae)	Severity of sequelae	Availability of treatment/ vaccine
Leptospira spp.	1% (WHO 2003) 14% (Costa *et al.* 2001) 22% in Italy (Ciceroni *et al.* 2000)	Elderly at higher risk than young, 11–47% in special groups (Lopez *et al.* 2001).	10 per 10,000 cases (WHO 2003) 30–50% (Smythe *et al.* 2000; Sasaki *et al.* 1993)	10–20 days	5–24% develop aseptic meningitis (Arean 1962; De Brito *et al.* 1979)	May result in death	Antibiotic treatment available.
Mycobacterium avium	Low	AIDS patients very susceptible. Afessa (2001) 6% case-fatality rate for MAC in AIDS patients.	No data found, estimate <1%	No data found estimate, 8–16 days	No data found	Interferes with daily life	Combination of treatments often required due to ability of MAC to become drug resistant.
S. typhi	3.5% (WHO 2003) <1% with appropriate treatment (WHO 2003)	No data found but case-fatality rates are higher in children less than one year old and the elderly (Agarwal *et al.* 2004)	75% (New Zealand Food Safety Authority 2001)	3–4 weeks	2% develop arthritis (CDC 2004a) 0.5–5% develop perforation of the bowel (van Basten and Stockenbrugger 1994) 10–15% of those who have been ill for more than two weeks develop complications (Parry *et al.* 2002)	Interferes with daily life	Vaccination Treatment including chemotherapy, antibiotics.

Pathogenic agent	Case-fatality rate (%) in immunocompetent patients	Case-fatality rate (%) in immunocompromised / sensitive groups	Severity of acute illness (Median % requiring hospitalisation)	Duration of acute illness	Frequency of sequelae (% of cases developing sequelae)	Severity of sequelae	Availability of treatment/ vaccine
Shigella spp.	0.2% (Gerba *et al.* 1996) 0.16% (New Zealand Food Safety Authority 2001)	No data found. However, most deaths due to *Shigella* occur in the very young (60% in under fives) or the elderly (Clemens *et al.* 1999); 11% in malnourished children (Bennish and Wojtyniak 1991)	13.9% (New Zealand Food Safety Authority 2001)	Average 4–7 days	5–10% develop HUS (foodborne illness.com) Reactive arthritis 0.2–2.4% (Lindsay 1997)	May result in death	Antibiotic treatment available.
Vibrio vulnificus	50% (Tacket *et al.* 1984) 7–25% wound infections (Levine *et al.* 1993)	50% (Lerstloompleephunt *et al.* 2000)	91% (New Zealand Food Safety Authority 2001)	3–7 days	50% develop bloodstream infections	Can result in death	Antibiotic treatment. Surgical removal of infected limb may be required.

Table 3.5 Summary of data used to compile severity scores (protozoa and trematodes).

Pathogenic agent	Case-fatality rate (%) in immunocompetent patients	Case-fatality rate (%) in immunocompromised / sensitive groups	Severity of acute illness (Median % requiring hospitalisation)	Duration of acute illness	Frequency of sequelae (% of cases developing sequelae)	Severity of sequelae	Availability of treatment/ vaccine
C. parvum	0.001% (in the Milwaukee outbreak – Havelaar and Melse 2003) Low (WHO 2002)	19% (Connolly et al. 1988); 46% in AIDS patients (Fayer and Ungar 1986; 61% (CDC 1986)	15% - based on Milwaukee outbreak (New Zealand Food Safety Authority 2001) 13% (Craun et al. 1998)	2–3 weeks	Very small	Interferes with daily life	Limited treatment available.
Giardia duodenalis	0.1% (Hunter and Fewtrell 2001)	No data found	13% (Lopez et al. 1980)	3 days – several weeks	50–67% (Gerba et al. 1996)	Interferes with daily life	Chemotherapy available
Naegleria fowleri	High, recovery rare	No data found but very high	No data found, likely to be close to 100%	1 week – 10 days	No data found, estimate 10–20%	PAM results in almost 100% case-fatality rate (Anonymous 2002)	Antibiotic treatment available, but ineffective.
Schistosomiasis	0.0075% (15,000 deaths out of 200 million infected persons worldwide; WHO 2003)	No data found	No data found, estimate 5–10%	Weeks to months	10% (WHO 2003)	Progression of liver, kidney, or other dysfunction may occur for many years after transmission has been interrupted	Chemotherapy available.

Table 3.6 Summary of data used to compile severity scores (viruses).

Pathogenic agent	Case-fatality rate (%) in immuno-competent patients	Case-fatality rate (%) in immunocompromised / sensitive groups	Severity of acute illness (Median % requiring hospitalisation)	Duration of acute illness	Frequency of sequelae (% of cases developing sequelae)	Severity of sequelae	Availability of treatment/vaccine
Adenovirus	No data found, estimate 0.001–0.002%	48% (Hierholzer 1992)	Infection with type 4 and type 5 result in 25% hospitalisations	Pharyngoco-njunctival fever 1–4 weeks	No data found, estimate <1%	May result in death	No specific treatment.
Coxsackievirus	No data found, estimate <0.001%	No data found but the elderly, the very young and the immunocompromised are at greater risk of becoming seriously ill and dying. (Crabtree 1996)	No data found, estimate 5–10%	No data found, estimate three weeks	No data found, estimate <1%	May result in death	No specific treatment.
Echovirus (aseptic meningitis)	No data found, estimate <0.001%	Death occurred in 33–50% of patients with primary antibody deficiency exposed to enteroviral infection, primarily echovirus 11 (Halliday *et al.* 2003)	Aseptic meningitis, 87% (Gosbell *et al.* 2000)	No data found, estimate three weeks	No data found, estimate <1%	May result in death	No specific treatment.

Pathogenic agent	Case-fatality rate (%) in immuno-competent patients	Case-fatality rate (%) in immunocompromised / sensitive groups	Severity of acute illness (Median % requiring hospitalisation)	Duration of acute illness	Frequency of sequelae (% of cases developing sequelae)	Severity of sequelae	Availability of treatment/ vaccine
Viral hepatitis caused by HAV	2% (Khauroo 2003) 0.6% (adults) (Gerba et al. 1996)	1.8% among adults >50 years of age; persons who have chronic liver disease have a high risk of death from fulminant HAV (Akriviadis and Redeke 1989; Lemon and Shapiro 1994) 1.5 per 1000 in children <5 years of age (HepNet 2000)	13% (New Zealand Food Safety Authority 2001)	Several weeks – months	Very small	No disability or interference with daily life	Vaccination. Lifetime immunity after early life exposure.

Table 3.7 Severity index applied to selected bacterial pathogens which may be transmitted through recreational waters.

Pathogen	CFR* Score	Acute severity score	Acute duration Score	Severity of sequelae score	Frequency of sequelae score	Final score for immuno-competent	Final score for immuno-compromised (where data is available)	Indication of prevalence or incidence
Camptylobacter spp.	1	1	2	2	2	8	13	15 cases per 100,000 per year in the United States (CDC 2003b)
Shiga toxin-producing *E. coli*	1	5	2	3	2	13	Insufficient data	73,000 cases of *E. coli* O157 annually in the United States (CDC 2004a)
Helicobacter pylori	3	1	3	3	4	14	Insufficient data	High (50–60% worldwide), responsible for 80% of stomach ulcers (Duck *et al.* 2004)
Legionella spp. (causing Legionnaires disease)	6	3	3	3	3	18	18	Between 8000 and 18,000 cases of Legionnaires' disease in the United States annually (CDC 2004c)
Leptospira spp.	6	3	4	3	3	19	19	Low, but under reported (Bharti *et al.* 2003) 100–200 cases per year in the United States (Farr 1995)

Pathogen	CFR* Score	Acute severity score	Acute duration Score	Severity of sequelae score	Frequency of sequelae score	Final score for immuno-competent	Final score for immuno-compromised (where data is available)	Indication of prevalence or incidence
Mycobacterium avium	1	1	4	1	1	8	11	Incidence between 1 and 2.5 per 100,000 (Marras and Daley 2002)
Salmonella typhi	2	5	5	1	2	15	Insufficient data	In the United States about 400 cases occur each year, and 70% of these are acquired while travelling internationally. Typhoid fever affects about 12.5 million persons each year in the developing world (CDC 2004b).
Shigella spp.	1	2	2	3	2	11	15	18,000 cases reported annually in the United States. Actual figure likely to be considerably higher (CDC 2003c)
Vibrio vulnificus (septic wound infections)	6	5	2	3	5	21	21	Low, but under-reported

* CFR; case-fatality rate

Table 3.8 Severity index applied to selected protozoans and trematodes which may be transmitted through recreational waters.

Pathogen	CFR* Score	Acute severity score	Acute duration Score	Severity of sequelae score	Frequency of sequelae score	Final score for immuno-competent	Final score for immuno-compromised (where data is available)	Indication of prevalence or incidence
Cryptosporidium parvum	1	4	5	1	1	12	17	1.17 in 100,000 people infected in the United States although much higher based on serological studies (Groseclose *et al.* 2002)
Giardia duodenalis	1	4	3	1	5	14	Insufficient data	Prevalence varies between 3% in developed countries (Farthing 1994) and 20% in developing countries (Islam 1990)
Naegleria fowleri	6	5	4	3	4	22	Insufficient data	Low, 1–3 cases per year in the United States (Levy *et al.* 1998)
Schistosomiasis	1	3	5	3	2	14	Insufficient data	200 million people infected worldwide, but in specific regions only (WHO 2003)

* CFR; case-fatality rate

Table 3.9 Severity index applied to selected viruses which may be transmitted through recreational waters.

Pathogen	CFR* Score	Acute severity score	Acute duration Score	Severity of sequelae score	Frequency of sequelae score	Final score for immuno-competent	Final score for immuno-compromised (where data is available)	Indication of prevalence or incidence
Hepatitis A	2	4	5	1	1	13	Insufficient data	1.5 million cases worldwide annually, serological evidence suggests 15–100% previous exposure, of particular concern for travellers from high sanitation to low sanitation environments (WHO 2003).
Echovirus	1	3	5	3	1	13	18	High – around 30 million cases in the United States (WHO 2004)
Coxsackievirus	1	3	5	3	1	13	Insufficient data	High
Adenovirus	1	5	5	3	1	15	20	High

* CFR; case-fatality rate

Table 3.10 Management strategies for controlling risks of severe disease outcomes associated with recreational water exposure.

Source of Pathogen	Examples of Pathogen	Management Strategies
Human Excreta*	*Salmonella typhi* *Shigella* spp. Hepatitis A Virus Hepatitis E Virus *Helicobacter pylori* *Schistosoma* spp.	Close recreational areas subject to combined sewer overflow discharges after heavy storm events Treat sewage to reduce pathogens prior to environmental discharge Vaccination Treatment of infected individuals Provide access to adequate sanitation facilities and safe drinking water
Animal Excreta*	*Cryptosporidium parvum* *Campylobacter* spp. *E. coli* O157 *Leptospira* spp.	Prevent livestock access to waterbodies Create vegetative buffer zones between farms and waterbodies Treat animal manures prior to land-application Use farming methods that reduce soil erosion and surface runoff Vaccinate domestic animals and livestock
Naturally Occurring	*Naegleria* *Mycobacterium avium* complex *Vibrio vulnificus*	Education of recreational water users and public health professionals Beach warnings Create disease surveillance mechanisms
Naturally Occurring Situation Specific	*Legionella* spp. *Naegleria*	Manage pools, spas, and water distribution networks appropriately Public education, post warning signs where conditions favour growth of amoeba

*Some pathogens may have both human and/or animal sources

The pathogens described in this review are not necessarily found in all locations and therefore the risk to recreational users will vary depending on location due to the probability of encountering the particular pathogen. Schistosomiasis for example, although found worldwide is most prevalent in sub-Saharan Africa, southern China, the Philippines, and Brazil.

For some of the pathogens included in this review the only reasonable option available to managers is to introduce risk communication in the recreational water area where the pathogen is known to reside. The severity index could be used to indicate the need to develop educational materials for susceptible sub-populations. For example, signs could be posted at recreational areas to warn immunocompromised individuals about possible hazards, especially if the water is prone to contamination from human or animal wastes during storm events. Or, doctors could be warned to look for specific diseases in vulnerable groups.

For others, wastewater treatment interventions would reduce the risk to recreational users. However, the costs may be prohibitive or may divert resources away from other priorities. Management recommendations to prevent the transmission of infectious diseases through water use are described in the WHO *Guidelines for Safe Recreational Water Environments*, volumes 1 and 2 (WHO 2003; WHO 2005).

3.5 SUMMARY

The use of water for recreational purposes poses a number of health risks which depend on factors such as the nature of the hazard, the characteristic of the water body and the immune status of the user. Although evidence from outbreak reports and other epidemiological evidence have proven a link between adverse health effects and immersion in poor quality recreational water, most illness is mild and self-limiting and not reported. Illnesses reported by surveillance systems are probably underestimates of illness associated with waterborne disease agents.

Even where illness is severe, it may still be difficult to attribute it to recreational water exposure due to the large number of other transmission routes of the pathogens in question. Nevertheless, evidence does exist to show that although much less frequent, more serious and potentially fatal disease is also a risk to recreational users of water.

REFERENCES

Afessa, B (2001) Mycobacterial and nonbacterial pulmonary complications in hospitalized patients with human immunodeficiency virus infection: A prospective, cohort study. *BMC Pulmonary Medicine*, **1**(1), 1.

Agarwal, P.K., Gogia, A. and Gupta, R.K. (2004) Typhoid fever. *Journal of Indian Academy of Clinical Medicine*, **5**(1), 60–64.

Akriviadis, E.A. and Redeker, A.G. (1989) Fulminant hepatitis A in intravenous drug users with chronic liver disease. *Annals of Internal Medicine*, **110**, 838–839.

Allos, B.M. and Blaser, M.J. (1995) *Campylobacter jejuni* and the expanding spectrum of related infections. *Clinical Infectious Diseases*, **20**, 1092–1099.

Anonymous (1996) Strength of association between human illness and water: revised definitions for use in outbreak investigations. *CDR Weekly*, **6**(8), 1.

Anonymous (1983) Epidemiologic notes and reports gastrointestinal illness among scuba divers – New York City. *MMWR*, **32**(44), 576–577.

Anonymous (2002) Primary amebic meningoencephalitis – Georgia, 2002. *MMWR*, **52**(40), 962–964.

Arean, V.M. (1962) The pathologic anatomy and pathogenesis of fatal human leptospirosis (Weils disease). *American Journal of Pathology,* **40,** 393-396.

Barbaro, G. (2002) Legionella. *The Lancet Infectious Diseases,* **2**(7), 447.

Bennish, M.L. and Wojtyniak, B.J. (1991) Mortality due to shigellosis: community and hospital data. *Reviews of Infectious Diseases,* **13**(4), S245–S251.

Bharti, A.R., Nally, J.E., Ricaldi, J.N., Matthias, M.A., Diaz, M.M., Lovett, M.A., Levett, P.N., Gilman, R.H., Willig, M.R., Gotuzzo, E., Vinetz, J.M., and Peru-United States Leptospirosis Consortium (2003). Leptospirosis: a zoonotic disease of global importance. *The Lancet Infectious Diseases,* **3**(12), 757–771.

Bohte, R., van Furth, R. and van den Broek, P.J. (1995) Aetiology of community-acquired pneumonia: a prospective study among adults requiring admission to hospital. *Thorax,* **50,** 543–547.

Buzby, J.C., Mishu Allos, B.M. and Roberts, T. (1997) The economic burden of *Campylobacter* associated Guillain-Barré syndrome. *Journal of Infectious Diseases,* **176**(2) 192–197.

Centers for Disease Control and Prevention (CDC) (1986) Classification system for human lymphotropic virus type III/ lympadenopathy-associated virus infections. *Morbidity and Mortality Weekly Report,* **35,** 334–339.

Centers for Disease Control and Prevention (CDC) (2003a) http://www.cdc.gov/ulcer/md.htm. Accessed 22 June 2005.

Centers for Disease Control and Prevention (CDC) (2003b) http://www.cdc.gov/ncidod/dbmd/diseaseinfo/campylobacter_g.htm#How%20common%20is%20Campylobacter. Accessed 22 June 2005.

Centers for Disease Control and Prevention (CDC) (2003c) http://www.cdc.gov/ncidod/dbmd/diseaseinfo/shigellosis_g.htm. Accessed 22 June 2005. Accessed 22 June 2005.

Centers for Disease Control and Prevention (CDC) (2004a) http://www.cdc.gov/ncidod/dbmd/diseaseinfo/escherichiacoli_g.htm. Accessed 22 June 2005.

Centers for Disease Control and Prevention (CDC) (2004b) http://www.cdc.gov/ncidod/dbmd/diseaseinfo/typhoidfever_g.htm. Accessed 22 June 2005.

Centers for Disease Control and Prevention (CDC) (2004c) http://www.cdc.gov/ncidod/dbmd/diseaseinfo/legionellosis_g.htm#How%20common%20is%20legionellosis%20in%20the%20United%20States. Accessed 22 June 2005.

Ciceroni, L., Stepan, E., Pinto, A., Pizzocaro, P., Dettori, G., Franzin, L., Lu Mansueto, S., Manera, A., Ioli, A., Marcuccio, L., Grillo, R. and Ciarrocchi, S. (2000) Epidemiological trend of human leptospirosis in Italy between 1994 and 1996. *European Journal of Epidemiology,* **16**(1), 79– 86.

Clemens, J., Kotloff, K. and Kay, B. (1999) Generic protocol to estimate the burden of *Shigella* diarrhoea and dysenteric mortality. Department of Vaccines and Biological, World Health Organization, Geneva.

Connolly, G.M., Dryden, M.S., Shanson, D.C. and Gazzard, B.G. (1988) Cryptosporidial diarrhoea in AIDS and its treatment. *Gut,* **29,** 593–597.

Costa, E., Costa, Y.A., Lopes, A.A., Sacramento, E. and Bina, J.C. (2001). Severe forms of leptospirosis: clinical, demographic and environmental aspects. *Revista da Sociedade Brasileira de Medicina Tropical,* **34**(3), 261–267.

Crabtree, K.D. (1996) Waterborne ritavirus and coxsackievirus: a risk assessment approach. Drinking Water and Health Newsletter, Chlorine Chemistry Council, Arlington, VA, USA. Available on-line: http://c3.org/news_center/ccc_periodicals/drinking_water/dwhn070196.html. Accessed 22 June 2005.

Craun, G.F., Berger, P.S. and Calderon, R.L. (1996) Coliform bacteria and waterborne disease outbreaks. *Journal of the American Waterworks Association*, **9**, 96–104.

Craun, G.F, Hubbs, S.A., Frost, F., Calderon, R.L. and Via, S.H. (1998) Waterborne outbreaks of cryptosporidiosis. *Journal of American Waterworks Association*, **90**, 81–91.

Craun, G.F., Nwachuku, N., Calderon, R.L. and Craun, M.F. (2002) Outbreaks in drinking-water systems, 1991–1998. *Journal of Environmental Health*, **65**, 16–25.

De Brito, T., Bohm, G..M. and Yasuda, P.H. (1979) Vascular damage in acute experimental leptospirosis of the guinea-pig. *Journal of Pathology*, **128**, 177-182.

Duck, W.M., Sobel, J., Pruckler, J.M., Song, Q., Swerdlow, D., Friedman, C., Sulka, A., Swaminathan, B., Taylor, T., Hoekstra, M., Griffin, P., Smoot, D., Peek, R., Metz, D.C., Bloom, P.B., Goldschmid, S., Parsonnet, J., Triadafilopolous, G., Perez-Perez, G.I., Vakil, N., Ernst, P., Czinn, S., Dunne, D. and Gold, B.D. (2004) Antimicrobial resistance incidence and risk factors among *Helicobacter pylori*-infected persons, United States. *Emerging Infectious Diseases*, **10**(6) 1088–1094.

Farr, R.W. (1995) Leptospirosis. *Clinical Infectious Diseases*, **21**, 1–8.

Farthing, M.J.G. (1994) Giardiasis as a disease. In: *Giardia: From molecules to disease*. (ed. R.C.A. Thompson, J.A. Reynoldson and A.J. Lymbery), pp. 15–37, Wallingford, CAB International, UK.

Fayer, R. and Ungar, B.L.P. (1986). *Cryptosporidium* spp. and cryptosporidiosis. *Microbiological Reviews*, **50**, 458–483.

Fleisher J.M., Kay D., Wyer M.D. and Godfree, A.F. (1998) Estimates of the severity of illnesses associated with bathing in marine waters contaminated with domestic sewage. *International Journal of Epidemiology*, **27**(4), 722–726.

Gerba, C.P., Rose, J.B. and Haas, C.N. (1996) Sensitive populations: who is at the greatest risk? *International Journal of Food Microbiology*, **30**, 113–123.

Gosbell, I., Robinson, D., Chant, K and Crone, S. (2000) Outbreak of echovirus 30 meningitis in Wingecarribee Shire, New South Wales. *Communicable Diseases Intelligence*, **24**(5), 121–124.

Groseclose, S.L., Braithwaite, W.L., Hall, P.A., Knowles, C., Adams, D.A., Connor, F., Hester, M., Sharp, P., Anderson, W.J. and Fagan, R.F. (2002) Summary of notifiable diseases – United States 2000. *MMWR*, **49**(53), 1–102.

Halliday, E., Winkelstein, J. and Webster, A.D.B. (2003) Enteroviral infections in primary immunodeficiency (PID): a survey of morbidity and mortality. *Journal of Infection*, **46**(1), 1–8.

Havelaar, A.H. and Melse, J.M. (2003). *Quantifying public health risks in the WHO Guidelines for Drinking-water Quality: a burden of disease approach.* Report 734301022/2003, RIVM, Bilthoven, Netherlands.

HepNet (2000) http://www.hepnet.com/hepc/aasld00/alter.html. Accessed 22 June 2005.

Hierholzer, J.C. (1992) Adenovirus in the immunocompromised host. *Clinics in Microbiological Reviews*, **5**, 262–274.

Hunter, P. and Fewtrell, L. (2001) Acceptable Risk. In: *Water Quality: Guidelines, Standards and Health,* (ed. L. Fewtrell and J. Bartram), IWA Publishing, UK on behalf of World Health Organization.

Hunter, P. and Nichols, G. (2002) Epidemiology and clinical features of Cryptosporidium infection in immunocompromised patients. *Clinical Microbiology Reviews*, **15**(1) 145–154.

Islam, A. (1990) Giardiasis in developing countries. In *Human parasitic diseases*, vol. 3, (ed. E.A. Meyer), pp. 235–266, Elsevier, Amsterdam, The Netherlands.

Khauroo, M.S. (2003) Viral hepatitis in international travellers: risks and prevention. *International Journal of Antimicrobial Agents,* **21**(2), 143–152.

Lansbury, L.E. and Ludlam, H. (1997). *Escherichia coli* O157: Lessons learnt from the past 15 years. *Journal of Infection,* **34**, 189–198.

Lemon S.M. and Shapiro C.N. (1994) The value of immunization against hepatitis A. *Infectious Agents of Disease,* **1,** 38–49.

Lerstloompleephunt, N., Tantawichien, T. and Sitprija, V. (2000) Renal failure in vibrio vulnificus infection. *Renal Failure,* **22**(3), 337–343.

Levine, W.C., Griffin, P.M., Woernle, C.H., Klontz, K.C., Maclafferty, L.L., Mcfarland, L.M., Wilson, S.A., Ray, B.J. and Taylor, J.P. (1993) Vibrio infections on the Gulf Coast – Results of first year of regional surveillance. *Journal of Infectious Diseases,* **167**, 479–483.

Levy, D.A., Bens, M.S., Craun, G.F., Calderon, R.L. and Herwaldt, B.L. (1998) Surveillance for waterborne-disease outbreaks – United States, 1995–1996. *MMWR,* **47**, 1–34.

Lindsay, J.A. (1997) Chronic sequelae of foodborne disease. *Emerging Infectious Diseases,* **3**(4), 442–452.

Lopez, A.A., Costa, E., Costa, Y.A., Bina, J.C. and Sacramento, E. (2001) The association between serum potassium at hospital admission and the case-fatality rate of leptospirosis in men. *Revista do Instituto de Medicina Tropical de Sao Paulo,* **43**(4), 217–220.

Lopez, C.E., Dykes, A.C., Juranek, D.D., Sinclair, S.P., Conn, J.M., Christie, R.W., Lippy, E.C., Schultz, M.G. and Mires, M.H. (1980) Waterborne giardiasis: a community wide outbreak of disease and a high rate of asymptomatic infection. *American Journal of Epidemiology,* **112**(4), 495–507.

Maggini, M., Salmaso, S., Alegiani, S.S., Caffari, B. and Raschetti, R. (1991) Epidemiological use of drug prescriptions as markers of disease frequency: an Italian experience. *Journal of Clinical Epidemiology,* **44**, 1299–1307.

Mandell, G.L., Douglas, R.G. and Bennett, J.E. (1990) *Principles and Practice of Infectious Diseases*. Churchill Livingstone, New York, United States.

Marras, T.K. and Daley, C.L. (2002) Epidemiology of human pulmonary infection with nontuberculous mycobacteria. *Clinics in Chest Medicine,* **23,** 553–567.

Miller, J.R., Ashendorf, A. Seeley, A., Mikol, Y.B., Faber Jr., W.W., Calder, J. and Layton, M. (1997) Descriptive epidemiology of cryptosporidosis in New York City. *International Symposium on waterborne Cryptosporidium proceedings*, (ed. C.R. Fricker, J.L. Clancy and P.A. Rochelee), pp. 317–328 American Water Works Association, Denver, Co.

Muder, R.R., Yu, V.L., and Fang, G.D. (1989) Community-acquired Legionnaires' disease. *Seminars in Respiratory Infections,* **4**, 32–39.

New Zealand Food Safety Authority (2001) *Microbial data sheets.* Available on-line. http://www.nzfsa.govt.nz/science-technology/data-sheets/. Accessed 22 June 2005.

Parry, C.M., Hien, T.T., Dougan, G., White, N.J. and Farrar, J.J. (2002) Typhoid fever. *The New England Journal of Medicine,* **347**(22), 1770–1782.

Proctor, M.E., Blair, K.A. and Davis, J.P. (1998) Surveillance data for waterborne illness detection: an assessment following a massive waterborne outbreak of *Cryptosporidium* infection. *Epidemiology and Infection,* **120**, 43–54.

Sasaki, D.M., Pang, L., Minette, H.P., Wakida, C.K., Fujimoto, W.J., Manea, S.J., Kunioka, R. and Middleton, C.R. (1993) Active surveillance and risk factors for leptospirosis in Hawaii. *American Journal of Tropical Medicine and Hygiene,* **48**(1), 35–43.

CAMPYLOBACTER

Credibility of association with recreational water: Probably associated

I Organism

Pathogen

Campylobacter spp.

Taxonomy

Gram-negative, non-spore forming, curved, S-shaped or spiral rods belonging to the family Campylobacteraceae. There are 15 species associated with the genus *Campylobacter*. The organisms are slender, spirally-curved Gram-ngative rods.

Reservoir

Most species of *Campylobacter* are adapted to the intestinal tract of warm-blooded animals. It is thought that a large number of gulls carry *Campylobacter* spp. (Levesque *et al.* 2000). The large reservoir in animals, particularly poultry is probably the ultimate source for most infections in humans (Park 2002).

Distribution

Worldwide.

Characteristics

Campylobacter appear in a variety of environments. *Campylobacter* has been shown to be able to enter a viable but dormant state to overcome adverse conditions (Talibart *et al.* 2000). The organisms grow optimally in the laboratory in atmospheres containing 5% oxygen. They have a restricted temperature growth range, growing optimally at 42°C and do not grow at temperatures below 30°C, unless associated with amoeba (Axelsson-Olsson *et al.*, 2005). They do not survive in dry conditions and are sensitive to osmotic stress (Park 2002).

II Health aspects

Primary disease symptoms and sequelae

C. jejuni and *C. coli* are a major cause of acute enterocolitis in humans. *C. enteritis* is the most common form of infective diarrhoea in most developed countries of the world (Skirrow 1991). *C. jejuni* has been reported to produce a cholera-like enterotoxin (Calva *et al.* 1989). Most symptomatic infections occur in infancy and early childhood. Clinical symptoms of *C. jejuni* infection are characterised by cramps, abdominal pain, diarrhoea (with or without blood or faecal leukocytes), chills and fever, which are self-limited and resolve in three to seven days. Relapses may occur in 5% to 10% of untreated patients.

Most infections do not require treatment. However, treatment with antibiotics does reduce the length of time that infected individuals shed the bacteria in their faeces.

Evidence shows an association of campylobacter infection with acute inflammatory demyelinating polyneuropathy – known as Guillain-Barré syndrome (Kaldor and Speed 1984; Winer *et al.* 1988). Approximately 1 in 1000 diagnosed infections leads to Guillain-Barré syndrome, a paralysis that lasts weeks to months and usually requires intensive care. Approximately 5% of patients with Guillain-Barré syndrome will die (Alketruse *et al.* 1999). Although rare, a number of cases are described in the literature (see for example, Colle *et al.* 2002; Kuwabara *et al.* 2002). It begins several weeks after the diarrhoeal illness in a small minority of campylobacter victims. Guillain-Barré syndrome occurs when a person's immune system makes antibodies to campylobacter and these antibodies attack components of the body's nerve cells because they are chemically similar to bacterial components. Guillain-Barré syndrome begins in the feet and spreads up the body. Prickling sensations lead to weakness that may lead to paralysis. It lasts for weeks to months and often requires intensive care. Full recovery is common, however victims may be left with severe neurological damage and many patients are left with residual signs such as loss of strength and fatigue and in some cases loss of libido. Approximately 15% of people with Guillain-Barré syndrome remain bedridden or wheelchair-bound at the end of one year (Bernsen *et al.* 2002).

Studies have also shown an association between infection with campylobacter and acute motor neuropathy, particularly in northern China, although it may occur in other parts of the world (Wirguin *et al.* 1997).

Miller Fisher syndrome is another, related, neurological syndrome that can follow campylobacteriosis and is also caused by immunologic mimicry. In Miller Fisher syndrome, the nerves of the head are affected more than the nerves of the body. Kuroki *et al.* (2001) have reviewed three cases of ophthalmoplegia associated with *C. jejuni*.

A fourth chronic condition that may be associated with campylobacter infection is an arthritis called Reiter's syndrome. This is a reactive arthritis that most commonly affects large, weight-bearing joints such as the knees and the lower back. It is a complication that is strongly associated with a particular genetic make-up; persons who have the human lymphocyte antigen B27 (HLA-B27) are most susceptible. Reactive arthritis following infection has been reported in numerous case reports or series and was recently reviewed by Nachamkin (2002) and Skirrow and Blaser (2000).

Campylobacter may also cause appendicitis or infect the abdominal cavity (peritonitis); the heart (carditis); the central nervous system (meningitis); the gallbladder (cholecystitis); the urinary tract and the blood stream (Ang *et al.* 2001). It can cause life-threatening sepsis in persons with compromised immune systems. Other clinical manifestations of *C. jejuni* infections in humans include septic arthritis, meningitis and protocolitis secondary to *C. jejuni.*

Fatality from *C. jejuni* generally only occurs in infants, elderly individuals, and patients with significant co-morbidities (Alketruse *et al.* 1999). However there has been at least one reported maternal fatality, secondary to shock and respiratory failure, occurring 11 days after the death of the foetus and 17 days after the onset of symptoms (McDonald and Gruslin 2001).

Exposure/mechanism of infection

Infection occurs through the consumption of infected meat or through water contaminated with the excreta of infected animals. Faecal–oral or person-to-person transmission of *C. jejuni* has been reported. The initial site of colonisation is the upper small intestine. *C. jejuni* multiplies in human bile. The bacteria colonises the jejunum, ileum, and colon (Mandell *et al.* 1990).

Disease incidence

Even though surveillance is very limited, it is thought that campylobacter is the leading cause of acute infectious diarrhoea in most industrialised countries (McDonald and Gruslin 2001). The incidence of *C. enteritis* differs from country to country and even among different regions of the same country, and has seasonal peaks in spring and summer (Skirrow 1990). Virtually all cases occur as isolated, sporadic events, not as a part of large outbreaks. Over 10,000 cases are reported to the United States CDC each year, equalling approximately six reported cases for each 100,000 persons in the United States population. Many more cases go undiagnosed or unreported. In the United States, disease caused by *C. jejuni* or *C. coli* has been estimated to affect seven million people annually, causing between 110 and 511 deaths and costing between $1.2 and $6 billion (Buzby and Roberts 1997).

The campylobacter sentinel surveillance scheme of England and Wales reported 7360 laboratory confirmed cases of campylobacteriosis in the year that it was established (CDSC 2000a). Of these 3% had consumed river, stream or spring water although it does not specify whether this was during the course of recreational activities. In this first year of surveillance reported cases were ill for a total of 79,090 days (mean 11 days) and 732 patients (10% of the total) required admission to hospital for at least 3048 days (mean five days). There were 5107 cases off work or unable to undertake their normal activities for a total of 38,769 days (mean eight days) (CDSC 2000a).

Incubation period

The incubation period for the diarrhoeal disease is usually two to four days (Hunter 1998).

Infectivity

Human volunteer studies have shown that the infective dose is between 500 organisms (Robinson 1981; Park 2002) and 1000 (WHO 2004a), although most natural infections probably require at least 10^4 organisms (Hunter 1998).

Sensitive groups

Campylobacter cases with AIDS have been shown to have higher rates of bacteremia and hospitalisation than *Campylobacter* cases without AIDS (Sorvillo *et al.* 1991). Human immunodeficiency virus also predisposes to recurrent infection. Fatality from *C. jejuni* generally only occurs in infants, elderly individuals, and patients with significant co-morbidities (Alketruse *et al.* 1999).

III Evidence for association of campylobacter with recreational waters

C. jejuni is one of the most common causes of bacterial gastroenteritis and chronic sequelae (Nachamkin 2002) and has been increasingly found in sewage and isolated from surface waters on many occasions (Lambert *et al.* 1998; Pianetti *et al.* 1998; Eyles *et al.* 2003) including from EU bathing waters (Brennhovd *et al.* 1992; Arvanitidou *et al.* 1995). This is not surprising since many domestic animals and waterfowl have been shown to shed this pathogen in their faeces contributing to the microbiological degradation of recreational waters (Levesque *et al.* 2000; WHO 2004a). In addition, any water that has been contaminated with human wastes has the potential to contain *C. jejuni* (Arvanitidou *et al.* 1995).

C. *lari* is also reported to be a causal agent of gastroenteritis (Mishu *et al.* 1992) and waterborne outbreaks have been attributed to it (Broczyk *et al.* 1987). Obiri-Danso and Jones (2000) isolated thermophilic camplyobacter (*C. lari* and urease positive thermophilic campylobacters) in intertidal sediments on three EU bathing beaches in the United Kingdom. Counts were higher in winter months. A similar seasonal pattern was found by Jones *et al.* (1990) who investigated campylobacter counts in seawater in Morecambe Bay – an EU designated bathing beach in the United Kingdom. *Campylobacter* spp. was thought not to survive for more than a few hours in the winter and for only a few minutes in the summer (Obiri-Danso and Jones 1999). However, there is evidence to suggest that *Campylobacter* spp. can survive in a viable but non-culturable form under adverse environmental conditions (Rollins and Colwell 1986). Beach sediment may therefore act as a reservoir for campylobacters in winter months.

No cases of illness from campylobacter associated with recreational waters were recorded by the CDC surveillance system between 1986 and 2002. In March 1999, an outbreak of *C. jejuni* was associated with a private pool in Florida, United States that did not have continuous chlorine disinfection and reportedly had ducks swimming in the pool (Lee *et al.* 2000a). Lund (1996) showed that *C. jejuni* is more sensitive to chlorine than most other waterborne pathogens and *E. coli*, indicating that it may easily be controlled in swimming pools by present disinfection practices.

IV Conclusions

Campylobacter spp. have been isolated from recreational waters on many occasions. However, few cases of illness have been reported through this route. Recreational waters exposed to animal and human waste are most likely to be contaminated with campylobacter.

Campylobacter spp.	Epidemiological evidence linking recreational water use with illness	Evidence from outbreak data of illness associated with recreational water	Documented cases of illness associated with recreational water	Documented cases of sequelae (in any situation)
	√	√	√	√

E. COLI O157

Credibility of association with recreational water: Strongly associated

I Organism

Pathogen

E. coli O157.

Taxonomy

E. coli belongs to Family Enterobacteriaceae. The family consists of 15 genera, each are classified by serotyping its H and O antigens. Most of the *E. coli* that are found in the human intestine are harmless but five pathogenic groups of *E. coli* cause disease in humans (Table 4.1).

Table 4.1 Pathogenic groups of *E. coli* causing disease in humans (Adapted from Kuntz and Kuntz 1999)

Classification of infection	Abbreviation	Main symptoms of infection
Enteroaggregative *E. coli*	EaggEC	Diarrhoea
Enterohaemorrhagic *E. coli*	EHEC	Diarrhoea, bloody diarrhoea, HUS, Thrombotic thrombocytopenic purpura (TTP)
Enteroinvasive *E. coli*	EIEC	Bloody diarrhoea
Enteropathogenic *E. coli*	EPEC	Diarrhoea
Enterotoxigenic *E. coli*	ETEC	Diarrhoea, Ileitis

Verocytotoxin-producing *E. coli* (or EHEC) produce potent toxins (verocytotoxin or Shiga-like toxin) and can cause severe disease in man (Clarke 2001). EHEC are responsible for a range of illnesses which may be severe and sometimes fatal, particularly in infants, young children and the elderly. Although EHEC strains are in a wide range of O serogroups, the most important one associated with human disease is O157. The significance of EHEC belonging to many of the other serogroups requires further evaluation (Kuntz and Kuntz 1999).

Verocytotoxin has been identified in stool samples from children with HUS, thus linking infection with EHEC to this life-threatening condition (Kuntz and Kuntz 1999).

prolonged periods, averaging 13 to 17 days compared with between six and eight days in adults (Armstrong *et al.* 1996). Children, therefore, pose a greater threat for transmission of organisms.

Disease incidence

Varies with age group, with the highest incidence of reporting occurring in children aged under 15 years (0.7 cases per 100,000 in the United States) (WHO 2005a) In the United States, *E. coli* O157 causes an estimated 250 deaths annually (Mahon *et al.* 1997).

Incubation period

The incubation period varies from one to eight days, average three to four days.

Infectivity

The infectious dose of *E. coli* O157:H7 is thought to be very low. Infection is linked to the consumption of less than 50 organisms and possibly as low as five (Armstrong *et al.* 1996).

Sensitive groups

Affects all ages, higher death rates occur in the elderly, immunocompromised and young (Health Canada 2001).

III Evidence for association of *E. coli* O157 with recreational waters

Studies have shown that *E. coli* O157:H7 is able to survive in a viable but non-culturable state in water (Wang and Doyle 1998). Several outbreaks of *E. coli* O157:H7 have been associated with recreational waters, particularly with swimming in freshwater ponds or wading pools (Levy *et al.* 1998; Wang and Doyle 1998). Those reported have identified patients with the development of HUS, highlighting the seriousness of this infection to users of recreational waters.

In the summer of 1991, 21 cases of *E. coli* O157:H7 were reported from people who had swum in a lake in Oregon, United States. Of these, seven were admitted to hospital and three developed HUS. Illness amongst swimmers was associated with swallowing the lake water. No specific source of infection was found and it was assumed that the source was other bathers (Keene *et al.* 1994).

In May 1992, six cases of infection with *E. coli* O157 phage type 49 were identified in a semi-rural area of Scotland, United Kingdom. One child developed HUS. Although the source of infection was not identified, available evidence indicated that a children's paddling pool was the centre of transmission of infection causing the outbreak (Brewster *et al.* 1994).

Between 1992 and 1999, 1333 cases of *E. coli* O157:H7 infection were reported to the Wisconsin Division of Public Health, United States. Of these 8.1% were related to recreational water (Proctor and Davis 2000).

Between 1995 and 1996, six outbreaks of gastroenteritis were found to be caused by *E. coli* O157 in the United States. In this same time-period WBDO were reported more frequently than in previous years and were associated primarily with recreational lake water (Levy *et al.* 1998).

In July 1995, 12 cases of *E. coli* O157 infection were identified in children who had visited an Illinois, United States, state park with a lake swimming beach. Seven cultures were confirmed *E. coli* O157:H7, three with positive serology, one with HUS and culture-confirmed *E. coli* O157, and one with culture-negative bloody diarrhoea. Two families each had two children with *E. coli* O157:H7. Bloody diarrhoea was experienced by nine cases; three cases developed HUS and were hospitalised for at least a month each. Case-control studies indicated that swimming at the park, taking lake water into the mouth and swallowing lake water were risk factors for illness (Anonymous 1996a).

Four children aged between 1.5 and 3.5 years were admitted to hospital in Rotterdam, The Netherlands, with HUS. All four had bathed in the same shallow lake within a period of five days along with several hundred other people who visited the lake each day. Patients suffered with diarrhoea for between 3 and 11 days after swimming and the first clinical signs of HUS developed six to seven days after the onset of diarrhoea. Although no O157:H7 DNA could be detected in lake water samples, the samples were taken 16 days after the latest possible date of contamination of the patients and it is thought that the micro-organism would no longer be viable (Cransberg *et al.* 1996).

Hildebrand *et al.* (1996) report that six children were infected with *E. coli* O157:H7 in an area of southwest London, United Kingdom, in summer 1993. Three children developed HUS and one died. Four of the six cases had visited an outdoor paddling pool which had no detectable chlorine levels in half of the water samples taken.

Friedman *et al.* (1999) report a cluster of gastrointestinal illnesses, including one case of HUS and one culture confirmed *E. coli* O157 infection, after a pool party in a park in Atlanta, Georgia, United States. Following interview of a cohort of people attending the party and park residents, 18 developed a gastrointestinal illness, including ten who met the definition of primary case (the first gastrointestinal illness within a household between defined dates in which the titre of IgG antibodies to *E. coli* O157 was elevated). After pool exposure was controlled for, no other exposure was significantly associated with primary illness. It was revealed that the pool had not been adequately chlorinated.

Seven children and one adult were infected by *E. coli* O157 after swimming in a public pool in the North-West of England in September 2004. The outbreak happened when the pool's chlorine levels dropped due to a blocked pump (Henry and Chamber 2004).

IV Conclusions

Although most outbreaks have been associated with food, a number of outbreaks have been reported from recreational use of waters, particularly in pools that were not adequately chlorinated. HUS with possible long-term sequelae is evident in between 2% and 8% of cases although no follow-up studies appear to have been conducted in people who contracted the infection from recreational water use. The acute disease tends to be moderately severe and of moderate duration.

E. coli O157:H7	Epidemiological evidence linking recreational water use with illness	Evidence from outbreak data of illness associated with recreational water	Documented cases of illness associated with recreational water	Documented cases of sequelae (in any situation)
	√	√	√	√

HELICOBACTER PYLORI

Credibility of association with recreational water: Possibly associated

I Organism

Pathogen

Helicobacter pylori.

Taxonomy

H. pylori are small microaerophilic, Gram negative, curved, microaerphilic bacteria. *H. pylori* is the type species of the genus *Helicobacter*. This genus originally contained two species – *H. pylori*, the human gastric pathogen, and *H. mustelae*, found in the stomach of ferrets. There are now at least 14 species in the genus. Two have been associated with gastric disease in humans – *H. pylori* and *H. heilmanii.*

Reservoir

Humans are the natural hosts of *H. pylori*. It was first isolated in 1982 from specimens of human gastric mucosa by Warren and Marshall (1984).

Distribution

The bacteria *H. pylori* is found worldwide.

Characteristics

H. pylori is found in the interface between the gastric epithelial cell surface and the overlying mucus layer (Carroll *et al.* 2004). Genotyping studies have shown that almost every *H. pylori*-positive person has an individually distinguishable strain (Kuipers *et al.* 2003).

II Health aspects

Primary disease symptoms and sequelae

Most *H. pylori* infections are chronic and result in an asymptomatic superficial gastritis. Once established the organism persists in most individuals for many years. Infection with *H. pylori* has been linked to chronic gastrointestinal disease such as duodenal ulceration. Infection with *H. pylori* increases the risk of gastric or duodenal ulceration by about 50 times (Hunter 1998).

In developing countries *H. pylori* is acquired early in childhood, with infection rates of between 50% and 60% by the age of ten and up to 90% in adults (Megraud *et al.* 1989). By contrast in developed countries few infections occur in childhood and a gradual increase in prevalence is seen with age – with a rate of about 0.5–1% per year, leading to infection rates of between 20% and 30% by the age of 20 and of about 50% at 50 to 60 years. It is thought that a different degree of virulence, or the involvement of co-factors from the host or other bacteria in the host, are the reasons that most infected individuals are carriers of *H. pylori* and do not show any clinical symptoms (Dubois 1995).

Helicobacter spp. has been demonstrated in the liver of most patients with cirrhosis and hepatocellular carcinoma. *H. pylori* and related bacteria such as *H. hepaticus* produce toxins that kill the hepatocytes by a granulating effect on liver cell lines (Fagoonee *et al.* 2001).

Infection with *H. pylori* is associated with the development of gastric malignancies. Over 95% of patients with duodenal ulcers have *H. pylori* infection. The association between *H. pylori* and gastric ulcer is slightly less strong (Mou 1998). About 80% of patients with non-steroidal, anti-inflammatory drug-induced gastric ulcers have been infected. Several clinical reports have shown that *H. pylori* peptic gastric infection is a cause of refractory iron deficiency anaemia which does not respond to iron therapy and is not attributable to the usual causes (Barbarino 2002).

Epidemiological data suggests that *H. pylori* may be associated with non-Hodgkin's lymphoma and with mucosa-associated lymphoid tissue lymphoma (Parsonnet *et al.* 1996). In addition *H. pylori* may be associated with adenocarcinoma (Giesecke *et al.* 1993; Nguyen *et al.* 1999). Based on the evidence from a number of epidemiological studies which have shown a relationship between *H. pylori* and gastric cancer, the International Agency for Research on Cancer working group has classified *H. pylori* infection as a carcinogen (Laurila *et al.* 1999). Up to 15% (WHO 2003) of infected individuals develop the severe sequelae of gastric carcinoma or gastric lymphoma (Jones *et al.* 1999). Elimination of the bacterium may lead to an improvement in the histological appearance of the tumour (Hunter 1998).

The distribution of *H. pylori* infection and of its related diseases in various Asian countries is controversial. Although there is a strong link between *H. pylori* infection and gastric cancer in many countries, such as Japan, there is a large intercountry variation in incidence of gastric cancer and *H. pylori* seroprevalence among many Asian countries. For example, the prevalence of *H. pylori* infection is high in India and Bangladesh, but low gastric cancer rates have been reported. Factors that may influence the etiology of gastric cancer include the genetic diversity of the infecting *H. pylori* strains and differences in the host genetic background in various ethnic groups, including gastric acid secretion and genetic polymorphisms in proinflammatory cytokines. These factors, in addition to environmental factors, such as personal hygiene and dietary habits, reflect the multifactorial etiology of gastric cancer (Miwa *et al.* 2002).

There have been a number of reports of an association between *H. pylori* infection and non-gastrointestinal diseases. These include diabetes mellitus (Oldenburg *et al.* 1996); chronic headache (Gasbarrini *et al.* 1997; 1998; Realdi *et al.* 1999); skin disease (Wilson 1995; Murakami *et al.* 1996); autoimmune disorders (De Luis *et al.* 1998); and immunological disorders (Gasbarrini *et al.* 1998).

Realdi *et al.* (1999) and Strachan (1998) report an association between *H. pylori* and ischemic heart disease. Since the first report in 1994 until 1997, at least 20 epidemiological studies of about 2000 cases in total reported on the association of *H. pylori* antibody titres and human coronary heart disease or stroke. However, certain confounding factors such as socioeconomic status makes it difficult to say definitively from epidemiological studies whether a causal association exists (Danesh *et al.* 1997).

A few small studies report that individuals seropositive for *H. pylori* had high plasma concentrations or counts of some markers of inflammation that may also be associated with increased risks of vascular disease. However, apart from weak correlations with triglycerides and, inversely, with high-density lipoprotein cholesterol, no associations have been found between *H. pylori* and other vascular risk factors (Danesh *et al.* 1997).

A number of researchers have investigated the possible association between *H. pylori* infection and Sudden Infant Death Syndrome (Pattison *et al.* 1997; Rowland and Drumm 2001). However, Elitsur *et al.* (2000) and Ho *et al.* (2001) dispute this. This may not be surprising as Sudden Infant Death Syndrome is a disease of infants less than one-year-old whereas in developed countries infection with *H. pylori* is rarely seen in this age group. In developing countries where infection is seen in lower age groups the incidence of Sudden Infant Death Syndrome is low (Thomas *et al.* 1999).

Exposure/mechanism of infection

The exact mode of transmission is unclear but faecal–oral and oral–oral routes have been suggested (Velázquez and Feirtag 1999; Engstrand 2001). There have been a growing number of reports suggesting that water may be a route for spreading *H. pylori,* particularly in developing countries where management of water supplies is poor (Klein *et al.* 1991; Moreno *et al.* 2003), but in developed countries evidence supports the oral–oral transmission route (Hulten *et al.* 1996).

Disease incidence

Prevalence is assumed to be 50% worldwide (Carroll *et al.* 2004), with higher prevalence in developing than developed countries (Dunn *et al.* 1997). Rothenbacher and Brenner (2003) report prevalence in developing countries to be very high, with almost all children being infected by a certain age (possibly due to lower standards of personal hygiene; Parsonnet 1995), whereas the prevalence in developed countries seems considerably lower. Prevalence in adults ranges from 10% to 50% in the developed world and up to between 80% and 90% in the developing world. It is now thought that prevalence is declining.

In adults of industrialized countries, an estimated 0.5% of the susceptible population becomes infected each year. This incidence has been decreasing over time. Thus, adults who currently harbour the organism are more likely to have been infected in childhood than adulthood. The incidence of *H. pylori* infection is between 3% and 10% per year in developing countries.

Incubation period

Unknown.

Infectivity

Based on infection in Rhesus Monkeys, it is estimated that 10^4 bacteria are needed to infect specific-pathogen (*H. pylori*)-free monkeys (Solnick *et al.* 2001).

Sensitive groups

A number of determinants of more severe outcomes of the infection have been identified. Age of acquisition of *H. pylori* infection is thought to be one of these. Blaser *et al.* (1995) showed that men who acquired the infection early had an increased rate of gastric cancer and gastric ulcer but not duodenal ulcer. This implicates that gender is potentially a host factor predisposing to acquisition of the infection.

III Evidence for association of *Helicobacter pylori* with recreational waters

A number of studies have demonstrated that *H. pylori* survives in water and in biofilms (Mazari-Hiriart *et al.* 2001) although isolation of *H. pylori* from water systems has been shown to be difficult and there has been only one *in vivo* isolation of *H. pylori* from an environmental water source (Lu *et al.* 2002). When *H. pylori* is exposed to variable environmental conditions, changes in morphology, metabolism and growth patterns are observed resulting in a viable but non culturable (VNC) coccoid state (Graham *et al.* 1991; Bode *et al.* 1993). Shahamat *et al.* (1993) has shown that the VNC form in water is especially viable at temperatures between 4 °C and 15 °C. Virulence of this VNC state has also been proved (Aleljung *et al.* 1996; Wang *et al.* 1997).

The survival capacity of these organisms in surface water has been found to be between 20 and 30 days (Hegarty *et al.* 1999). *H. pylori* is readily inactivated by chlorine – however, substandard municipal water supplies may be a source of *H. pylori* infection.

H. pylori has been detected in well water, municipal water and treated water in Sweden (Hulten *et al.* 1998). Mazari-Hiriart *et al.* (2001) isolated *H. pylori* from canal water and surface water which children use for swimming in Xochimilco, Mexico. Goodman *et al.* (1996) report a study from children in an Andean community which found infection with *H. pylori* was more common in those who had swum in rivers, streams or in a swimming pool.

Apart from these cases no other published cases of infection with *H. pylori* attributed to recreational waters were found in the literature, although Mazari-Hiriart *et al.* (2001) and Frenck and Clemens (2003) support the theory that water could be one source of *H. pylori* infection, especially where water is not adequately treated. More and more numerous reports show that *H. pylori* DNA can be amplified from faeces samples of infected patients, which strongly suggests faecal–to–oral transmission. Therefore, it is possible that *H. pylori* infection is waterbome, but these assumptions need to be substantiated (Leclerc *et al.* 2002).

IV Conclusions

Water has been implicated as one mode of transmission of *H. pylori* although the detection of the pathogen has proved difficult. Therefore, it is possible that *H. pylori* infection is waterborne, but these assumptions need to be substantiated. Current evidence for its association with recreational waters is slight.

Helicobacter pylori	Epidemiological evidence linking recreational water use with illness	Evidence from outbreak data of illness associated with recreational water	Documented cases of illness associated with recreational water	Documented cases of sequelae (in any situation)
	None	None	√	√

LEGIONELLA

Credibility of association with recreational water: Strongly associated

I Organism

Pathogen

Legionellae.

Taxonomy

The legionellae consist of a single taxonomic group of related organisms comprising the family Legionellaceae, containing the genus *Legionella*. Two other genera have been proposed – *Fluoribacter,* containing *L. bozemanii* or *L. dumoffii,* and *Tatlockiea,* containing *L. micdadei*. At least 42 species of *Legionella* have been described (WHO 2004a).

L. pneumophila serogroup 1 is the type species and most frequently associated with Legionnaires' disease (Molmeret *et al.* 2001). Twenty species of legionella have been associated with human disease (Table 4.2).

Reservoir

Legionella spp. are naturally occurring aquatic organisms which have been isolated from natural freshwaters, including rivers, streams and lakes ranging in temperature up to 60 °C. They have also been isolated from waters in human environments polluted by man such as sewage-contaminated waters (Fewtrell *et al.* 1994).

Distribution

Distribution is worldwide but variations of the species/serogroups have been noted in a number of countries at different times (Bhopal 1993).

In 1988, *L. micdadei* accounted for the majority of cases of legionellosis reported in Victoria, Australia. In the United States, New Zealand and New South Wales, *L. micdadei* has been the most common non-pneumophila species implicated. In South Australia in 1988, of a total of 26 cases of legionellosis, *L. longbeachae* was identified in 20 and *L. pneumophila* in 6. In Victoria, Australia, of the 53 cases of legionellosis reported in the years 1983 to 1988, *L. pneumophila* was implicated in 40 cases and *L. micdadei* in 10 (Bhopal 1993).

Table 4.2 Species of legionella associated with disease in humans (adapted from Hunter 1998; Surman *et al.* 2005)

Species	Serogroup
L. anisa	
L. birminhamensis	
L. bozemanii	2
L. cincinnatiensis	
L. dumoffii	
L. erythra	
L. feeleii	
L. gormanii	
L. hackeliae	2
L. jordanis	
L. lansingensis	
L. longbeachae	2
L. macaechernii	
L. micdadei	
L. oakridgensis	
L. parisiensis	
L. pneumophila	16
L. sainthelensi	2
L. tusconensis	
L. wadsworthii	1

Characteristics

The legionellae can be distinguished from other bacteria by phenotypic and genetic properties – Gram-negative staining, non-fermentative metabolism, a requirement for growth *in-vitro* of L-cysteine and iron salts and the possession of branched chain cellular fatty acids. Legionellae are rod-shaped bacteria, 0.3–0.9 μ in width, and approximately 1.3 μ in length when grown *in vivo,* growing filaments up to 20 μ in length when grown *in vitro*. Significant multiplication of these bacteria occurs in the temperature range 25–50 °C (WHO 2004a).

Legionella bacteria have been shown to be very resistant to environmental factors. Long term persistence (up to ten years) of the same *L. pneumophila* serogroup 6 strain in a hospital water distribution system in France, and its association with sporadic cases of infection, has been reported (Lawrence *et al.* 1999).

Legionella bacteria will not grow in sterilised samples of the water from which they have been isolated. This suggests that they are part of a microbial ecosystem where they are nourished and protected. They are detected in higher numbers after other micro-organisms have developed and formed microbial communities in sediments, soils and biofilms. Fields (1993) has shown that in their natural habitat, freshwater and soil, growth of Legionella bacteria do require the presence of other bacteria or protozoa, which are considered to be natural hosts of legionellae. Uptake by ameoba such as *Naegleria fowleri* and survival of *L. pneumophila* is influenced by environmental conditions such as temperature (Newsome *et al.* 1985). The growth kinetics of *L. pneumophila* within ameoba such as *Acanthameoba* spp. and *Hartmannella* spp. vary according to the bacterial strain and factors such as the number of subcultures of the strain. Tison (1980) showed that *L. pneumophila* is significantly more stable when suspended in the fluid in which cyanobacteria had grown.

II Health aspects

Primary disease symptoms and sequelae

Legionnaires' disease (pneumonic legionellosis) is defined by the UK Health Protection Agency (http://www.hpa.org.uk) as a clinical diagnosis of pneumonia with microbiological evidence of infection with *L. pneumophila* serogroup 1, or a clinical diagnosis of pneumonia with microbiological evidence of infection with other *L. pneumophila* serogroups or other legionella species.

The term legionellosis includes Legionnaires' disease, which is a pneumonic illness, and non-pneumonic Pontiac fever. These are cases with microbiological evidence of legionella infection (confirmed or presumptive) and symptomatic respiratory illness but without evidence of pneumonia.

The first known infection with Legionnaires' disease was in 1957 in Minnesota, United States (Evenson 1998), but Legionnaires' disease first became publicly acknowledged in 1976 after an outbreak in Philadelphia, United States at an American Legion Convention in the Bellevue Stratford Hotel. A total of 221 cases of pneumonia and 34 deaths occurred. The outbreak was traced back to a cooling tower (Sanford 1979). Retrospective studies have shown that a number of outbreaks of pneumonia are now known to have been caused by legionella bacteria.

Typical symptoms of Legionnaires' disease are fatigue, fever, severe headache, muscle pain, chills, redness in the eyes, abdominal pain, jaundice, haemorrhages in the skin and mucous membranes, pneumonia, vomiting, severe prostration and mental confusion. The patient usually has a high temperature (102–105 °C). Diarrhoea is found in around 50% of patients and nearly 25% of patients show changes in mental status. Recovery is slow. Respiratory failure is a major cause of fatality in patients with Legionnaires' disease (Roig *et al.* 1993).

Sequelae include pericarditis (Ghannem *et al.* 2000), pleurisy (Taviot *et al.* 1987), myocarditis (Armengol *et al.* 1992), pyelonephritis, pancreatitis, and liver abscesses (Edelstein and Meyer 1984; Nguyen *et al.* 1991), empyema, pulmonary complications (Mamane *et al.* 1983), hypotension, shock, disseminated intravascular coagulation (Finegold 1988), thrombocytopenia (Larsson *et al.* 1999) and renal failure (Smeal *et al.* 1985). Andersen and Sogaard (1987) report evidence of cerebral abscess in a patient with serologically proven acute infection with legionella bacteria. Loveridge (1981) reports an association with arthritis, and seizures in patients with Legionnaires' disease have been reported by Peliowski and Finer (1986).

Exposure/mechanism of infection

Approximately 25% of cases of Legionnaires' disease are nosocomial in origin, the rest are community-acquired (Evenson 1998).

Legionella bacteria are thought to enter the lung via direct inhalation of aerosols. It is also thought that infection by aspiration following ingestion of contaminated water is common, particularly in people with damaged respiratory tracts, i.e. those with pre-existing lung disease or smokers. Once the bacterium enters the lung it replicates within alveolar macrophages until the cell ruptures and the bacteria are released into the lung where the cycle of multiplication continues.

There has been no proven person-to-person transmission of legionella bacteria although there was one suspected case in Glasgow, United Kingdom, in 1974. A general practitioner was treated for pneumonia. The clinical features suggested infection with *Mycoplasma pneumoniae*, *Chlamydia B* or *Coxiella burnetii*, but the serology was negative. The doctor himself was sure that he had contracted the infection from a patient whom he had seen two weeks before and had sent to hospital with severe pneumonia which had developed during a holiday abroad. Sera taken from the patient during his illness have proved, in retrospect, that he had Legionnaires' disease. No acute-phase serum was available from the general practitioner, but a sample taken more than three years later had an antibody of 1:512. This is strong circumstantial evidence of a case-to-case transmission (Love *et al.* 1978).

Disease incidence

Legionnaires' disease is thought to be the second most frequent cause of community-acquired pneumonia (Thi Minh Chau and Muller 1983). Helms *et al.* (1980) conducted an investigation in a rural community and found that serum antibodies against *L. pneumophila* serogroup 1 were found in 13.2% of the persons investigated. This suggests that infections with *L. pneumophila* are more frequent than estimated from outbreak reports. This could be due to misdiagnosis of flu-like symptoms and/or sub-clinical infection.

Outbreaks of Legionnaires' disease often receive significant media attention. However, this disease usually occurs as a single, isolated case not associated with any recognised outbreak. When outbreaks do occur, they are usually recognised in the summer and early autumn, but cases may occur year-round. Mortality is approximately 40% in patients with nosocomial infections and may be higher in immunosuppressed patients. Mortality from community-acquired infection ranges from 5% to 20% (Evenson 1998). In outbreaks of Pontiac fever attack rates up to 95% have been reported (Gotz *et al.* 2001).

An estimated 8000 to 18,000 people get Legionnaires' disease in the United States each year. Surveillance data from the CDC show that less than 10% of estimated cases are reported to local and state health officials (Anonymous 2004).

Surveillance data from Sweden record between 40 and 80 cases of Legionnaires' disease annually, half of them infected abroad (Gotz *et al.* 2001).

In Germany it is estimated that there are between 6000 and 7000 cases of pneumonia caused by legionella bacteria annually, with a death rate of between 15% and 20% (Thi Minh Chau and Muller 1983).

Between 1980 and 2000, 3,844 cases of Legionnaires' Disease were reported to the CDSC from residents in England and Wales; an average of 183 cases a year. Of these 43% of the cases were associated with travel abroad, 46% were community-acquired infections, 4% were associated with travel in the United Kingdom and 7% were linked to hospital-acquired infection (CDR 1991; Lee and Joseph 2002).

Incubation period

The incubation time for Legionnaires' disease is between three and six days (WHO, 2004a), although it may extend to ten days (Surman *et al.* 2005) but only one to two days for Pontiac fever. With Legionnaires' disease there is a sudden onset of symptoms.

Infectivity

The infective dose for humans is thought to be small – only a few or a single micro-organism. This is concluded from the fact that affected people are frequently found to have been exposed to contaminated aerosols generated at a considerable distance from them. In addition to the presence of a virulent micro-organism and a susceptible host, other unknown factors may be necessary for infection.

Sensitive groups

Legionnaires' disease usually affects individuals who are susceptible to the disease, i.e. the immunocompromised, typically smokers or those with lung or heart disease, and the elderly, males and alcoholics (Finegold, 1988; Nguyen *et al.* 1991). A person's risk of acquiring legionellosis following exposure to contaminated aerosols depends on a number of factors, including the nature and intensity of exposure and the exposed person's health status (Le Saux *et al.* 1989). Persons with chronic underlying illnesses, such as haematologic malignancy or end-stage renal disease, are at markedly increased risk for legionellosis (Bock *et al.* 1978; Kirby *et al.* 1980; Hoge and Breiman 1991). Persons in the later stages of AIDS are also probably at increased risk of legionellosis, but data are limited because of infrequent testing of patients. Nosocomial Legionnaires' disease has also been reported among patients at children's hospitals (Brady 1989).

Underlying disease and advanced age are not only risk factors for acquiring Legionnaires' disease but also for dying from the illness. In a multivariate analysis of 3524 cases reported to CDC between 1980 and 1989, immunosuppression, advanced age, end-stage renal disease, cancer, and nosocomial acquisition of disease were each independently associated with a fatal outcome (Marston *et al.* 1994). The mortality rate among 803 persons with nosocomially-acquired cases was 40% compared with 20% among 2721 persons with community-acquired cases (402), probably reflecting increased severity of underlying disease in hospitalised patients.

III Evidence for association of Legionnaires' disease with recreational waters

Most of the reported cases of Legionnaires' disease contracted from the recreational use of water are associated with the use of hot tubs (see below), although there are also a number of reported cases from the use of swimming pools and open waters.

Marine water is not a favourable environment for the growth of *Legionella* spp. It is suggested that sodium chloride is inhibitory to the growth of *L. pneumophila*. *L. pneumophila* are far more likely to be found in freshwaters especially where the temperature is higher. Legionellae tolerate chlorine much better than *E. coli* (Kuchta *et al.* 1983) and the resistance is further enhanced by inclusion in ameobae or by growth in biofilms, therefore disinfection of recreational waters with chlorine is not an effective method of protection. The resistance of Legionellae to ozone is comparable with that of *E. coli* or *Pseudomonas aeruginosa* (Domingue *et al.* 1988). Table 4.3 shows published reports of the occurrence of *Legionella* spp. in recreational waters.

Table 4.3 Reported occurrence of *Legionella* spp. in recreational waters.

Country	Reference	Notes
Bulgaria	Tomov *et al.* 1981	Isolation of legionella bacteria from a small mineral lake
Canada	Dutka and Evans 1986	Isolation of legionella bacteria from Canadian hot springs
United States	Cherry *et al.* 1982	*Legionella jordanis*: isolated from river water and sewage
United States	Palmer *et al.* 1993	Detection of *Legionella* spp. in sewage and ocean water
Puerto Rico	Ortiz-Roque and Hazen 1987	Abundance and distribution of *Legionella* spp. in Puerto Rican waters
Japan	Yabuuchi *et al.* 1994	*Legionella* spp. in hot spring bath water
Germany	Althaus 2000	*Legionella* spp. in drinking, bathing and warm water
Germany	Seidel 1987	Presence of *Legionella* spp. in water from warm spring pools
Italy	Leoni *et al.* 2001	Swimming pool water and showers showed signs of *Legionella* spp.
Italy	Martinelli *et al.* 2001	Water samples collected at three thermal spas
Italy	Sommese *et al.* 1996	Presence of *Legionella* spp. in thermal springs in Campania
Denmark	Jeppesen *et al.* 2000	*Legionella pneumophila* in pool water
England	Groothuis *et al.* 1985	*Legionella* spp. in hot tubs
Japan	Kuroki *et al.* 1998	Isolation of *Legionella* spp. at hot spring spas in Kanagawa, Japan
Japan	Kuroki *et al.* 1998	Occurrence of *Legionella* spp. in hot tubs

In Puerto Rico several species, including *L. bozemanii*, *L. dumoffii*, *L. gormanii*, *L. longbeachae*, *L. micdadei* and *L. pneumophila*, were found to be widely distributed in open waters, with the highest densities reported in sewage-contaminated waters (Ortiz-Roque and Hazen 1987).

Surveillance data

The European Surveillance Centres for Legionnaires' disease provided the following data concerning known cases of legionellosis associated with recreational waters.

Denmark

One case was reported by the Statensserum Institut, Department of Epidemiology. This was reported in January 1995, and a hot tub was the probable source of infection.

England and Wales

Laboratory surveillance data from England and Wales is available from 1980. A total of 29 cases of Legionnaires' disease and two cases of Pontiac fever were associated with recreational waters – all hot tubs – between 1980 and 2001 (Table 4.4).

Table 4.4 Outbreaks of Legionnaires' disease in England and Wales associated with recreational water activities 1980–2001 (Source: CDSC, England and Wales, personal communication).

Month/ year	Source	No. of cases	No. of deaths
May 1984	Hot tub	23 Legionnaires' disease	0
June 1992	Hot tub	One Legionnaires' disease and one Pontiac fever	0
August 1998	Hot tub	Five Legionnaires' disease and one Pontiac fever	1

Spain

Data was provided from 1993 to 2001. Table 3.5 provides details of cases of Legionnaires' disease associated with recreational waters reported to the Centro Nacional de Epidemiología, during this time period, together with the source of infection.

Table 4.5 Cases of Legionnaires' disease associated with recreational waters in Spain 1993–2001 (Source: Rosa Cano Portero, Sección de Información Microbiológica, Centro Nacional de Epidemiología, Spain, personal communication).

Micro-organism	Year	Cases	Deaths	Date of first case	Date of last case	Source of infection
L. pneumophila 1 Pontiac Philadelphia	1993	9	1	22/05/1993	02/06/1993	Hot spring/spa
L. pneumophila 2–14	1998	2	0	20/05/1998		Hot spring/spa
L. pneumophila 1	1999	11	0	20/05/1999		Spa
L. pneumophila Pontiac Knoxville	1999	11	0	1/04/1999	2/12/1999	Swimming pool
L. pneumophila 1	2000	3	0	4/08/2000	18/08/2000	Swimming pool/spa
L. pneumophila 1	2000	5	0	15/09/2000	13/10/2000	Swimming pool
L. pneumophila 1	2001	2	0	13/05/2001	26/05/2001	Swimming pool

Published cases of Legionnaires' disease associated with recreational waters

Published cases of Legionnaires' disease or Pontiac fever that are associated with recreational waters are shown in Table 4.6. Some specific cases are given in the following sections.

Table 4.6 Reported outbreaks of Legionnaires' disease or Pontiac fever associated with recreational waters.

Country	Reference	Notes
	WHO 1986	Legionnaires' disease associated with hot tub
	Vogt *et al.* 1987	Legionnaires' disease and hot tub
	Jernigan *et al.* 1996	Outbreak of Legionnaires' disease on cruise from spa use
	Den Boer *et al.* 1998	Legionnaires' disease and saunas
Australia	Anonymous 2000	Outbreak of Legionnaires' disease associated with aquarium
Denmark	Luttichau *et al.* 1998	Outbreak of Pontiac fever in children after hot tub use
Denmark	Luttichau *et al.* 1999	Pontiac fever following use of hot tub
France	Molmeret *et al.* 2001	Two cases of Legionnaires disease over three years associated with a thermal spa.
Japan	Tominaga *et al.* 2001	One case of Legionnaires' disease acquired from drinking hot spring water
Japan	IASR 2000	March 2000, 23 cases and 2 deaths from Legionnaires' disease June 2000, 43 cases and 3 deaths from Legionnaires' disease associated with bathing houses
Japan	Tokuda *et al.* 1997	Legionnaires' disease diagnosed in a man who drowned in public bath
Japan	Nakadate *et al.* 1999	An outbreak of Legionnaires disease associated with a spa
Japan	Kamimura *et al.* 1998	Legionella pneumonia caused by aspiration of hot spring water
Netherlands	Den Boer *et al.* 2002	133 confirmed and 55 probable cases of Legionnaires' disease acquired from display hot tub
United Kingdom (Scotland)	Goldberg *et al.* 1989 Fallon and Rowbotham 1990	Hot tub outbreak
Sweden	Gotz *et al.* 2001	Outbreak of Pontiac fever associated with a hotel hot tub
United Kingdom	McEvoy *et al.* 2000	Legionnaires' disease associated with exposure to a display hot tub

Country	Reference	Notes
United States	Mangione et al. 1985	Pontiac fever related to hot tub use
United States	Spitalny et al. 1984	Pontiac fever associated with hot tub use
United States	Spitalny et al. 1984	National survey on Legionnaires disease outbreaks associated with spas
United States	Benkel et al. 2000	23 laboratory-confirmed cases of Legionniares' disease associated with exposure to a display hot tub
United States	Fields et al. 2001	Pontiac fever from a hotel swimming pool and hot tub
United States	Tolentino et al. 1996	Hot tub legionellosis
United States	Jernigan et al. 1996	Legionnaires' disease on cruise ship – hot tub
United States	Mangione et al. 1985	Outbreak of Pontiac fever related to hot tub use, 14 people affected.
United States	Spitalny et al. 1984	Pontiac fever associated with hot tub.

Open waters

A review of the literature did not reveal any cases of Legionnaires' disease associated with marine water exposure. However, freshwater natural aquatic habitats are a possible source or reservoir of pathogenic *Legionella* spp.

Cases of Legionnaires' disease associated with hot springs/ hydrothermal areas

Hydrothermal areas are particularly suitable for the colonisation of *Legionella* spp. due to the warm water temperatures. Treatment is generally not allowed in thermal spas in order to preserve the characteristics of the mineral water.

Several studies have isolated *Legionella* spp. from spa waters (Bornstein et al. 1989; Shaffler-Dullnig et al. 1992; Mashiba et al. 1993; Martinelli et al. 2001). The large number of samples positive for legionella bacteria indicates a potential risk to users of thermal waters, especially those people that are undergoing inhalation treatment with thermal water, or those using hot tubs or taking a shower.

Nineteen aquatic sites from three hydrothermal areas on continental Portugal and one on the island of Sao Miguel, Azores, were tested for the presence of *Legionella* spp. Water temperatures varied between 22 °C and 67.5 °C, and the pH between 5.5 and 9.2. A total of 288 legionella isolates from 14 sites were identified. The majority of the isolates belonged to the species *L. pneumophila* (Verissimo et al. 1991).

Water samples from 66 thermal springs in the Campania region of southern Italy were cultured for *Legionella* spp. The temperature of the springs ranged from 21 °C to 59.5 °C. *L. pneumophila*, serogroups 7–10, was isolated from 2 out of 60 sources on the Island of Ischia and *L. dumoffii* from one mainland source. The temperatures of the sources were 35.2 °C, 48.2 °C and 52 °C, respectively (Sommese *et al.* 1996).

Shaffler-Dullnig *et al.* (1992) took water samples from hot water springs in an Austrian spa, as well as the water distribution system, and from various places of consumption of the thermal waters. Over 56% of the samples contained *L. pneumophila*; serogroups 1, 3, and 5 were most frequently identified. In this case no legionella bacteria was isolated from the inhalators in use.

A number of studies and cases of Legionnaires' disease have been reported from Japan. A province-wide survey of hot spring bath waters for the presence of *Legionella* spp. and free-living ameobae contamination was carried out by Kuroki *et al.* (1998). In a survey of 30 samples of hot spring baths from 12 sites in Kanagawa, Japan, *L. pneumophila* was detected in 21 water samples from 11 sites ranging from 10^1 to 10^3 cfu/100ml. *Naegleria* (46.7%), *Platyameoba* (33.3%), *Acanthameoba* (10.0%) and two other genera of free living ameobae were detected.

In 1993 a case of Legionnaires' disease was reported in Japan in a patient that had visited a hot (42 °C) spring. Water was collected from the bath as well as the shower and *L. pneumophila* serogroup 4 was isolated from the hot spring water, but not from the shower water. It was concluded that the patient's disease was contracted through aspiration of contaminated spring water (Mashiba *et al.* 1993).

Another case in Japan is reported of a man who was exposed to the sarin gas attack in the Tokyo subway in 1995, and visited a hot spring on the same day despite having symptoms such as tightness in the chest, headache, eye discomfort and muscle weakness. He developed difficulty breathing and was admitted to hospital where he died 71 days later. The post mortem revealed redness, edema and fragility of all visible areas of the airway, which was thought to be due to bronchitis caused by legionellosis (Kamimura *et al.* 1998).

A third case of Legionnaires' disease is reported from Japan by Yamauchi *et al.* (1998). This case was in a 54-year-old previously healthy woman who visited a hot spring spa. Ten days after visiting the hot spring she complained of lumbago, high fever and dry cough. She was admitted to hospital and was diagnosed with septic shock, disseminated intravascular coagulation and acute myocardial infarcation. Serum titre of *L. pneumophila* (serogroup 1) rose to 218-fold two weeks after the onset and legionella infection was highly suspected.

Two cases of Legionnaires' disease have been reported in people who visited the same thermal spa in France. The first was in 1994. A 40-year-old man with

Still's disease attended a 21-day thermal cure in a thermal spa in the Alpine region of France. Five days after returning home he developed severe acute pneumonia affecting both lungs. Clinical isolates of *L. pneumophila* were obtained by bronchoalveolar lavage. The man died four days after being admitted to hospital. The second case was a 69-year-old man with chronic obstructive bronchopneumonia who visited the spa in August 1997. He developed fever, cough and dyspnoea 15 days after arriving at the spa. X-ray revealed that he had pneumonia. He recovered after 20 days of antibiotics. To identify the source of the infection, 11 water samples were collected throughout the spa's distribution system. The thermal spa receives water from three natural springs and two bore holes. Water from the sources are then mixed and distributed throughout the spa's buildings at various temperatures which are optimal for the various uses/treatments. The 11 samples yielded 107 strains of legionella. Environmental samples were taken over a two-year-period. 81 strains were identified as *L. pneumophila* and 26 as *L. dumoffii*.

Two confirmed cases and six suspected cases of Legionnaires' disease were identified among people who were staying at a natural spa resort in Guipuzcoa, Spain between May 1 and May 22, 1999. *L. pneumophila* serogroup 1 was recovered from water samples taken at the spa resort which was closed following the discovery of the cases (Cano 1999).

Occurrence or likely occurrence of legionella in swimming pools

Legionella spp. have been isolated from swimming pool water on a number of occasions. Jeppesen *et al.* (2000) sampled water from 87 pools in Denmark of two temperatures (less than 28 °C and greater than 32 °C) and at various parts of the pools – from the bottom of the pool, the main body of the pool water and the water leaving from the activated carbon filters. Legionella bacteria was not detected in any of the samples from the colder pools but 10% of the warm water pool samples and 80% of the water from the filters contained legionella bacteria.

A similar study was carried out by Leoni *et al.* (2001) who sampled water from 12 indoor swimming pools in Bologna, Italy, four times in a year at a depth of 50 cm and at four different points one metre from the pool edge, giving a total of 48 samples. In addition, 48 samples of hot water were taken from the showers associated with the pools. Only two of the swimming pool samples were found to be positive for legionella bacteria whereas 27 of the samples from the showers were positive for legionella. Several species of legionella were isolated, indicating a widespread diffusion of these micro-organisms in the environment. Contamination by *L. pneumophila* found in some of the showers reached concentrations as high as 10^4 cfu/litre, which are levels similar to those found in other water systems during outbreaks of legionellosis (Patterson *et al.* 1994).

Cases of Legionnaires' disease associated with swimming pools

There are no reported cases of persons infected with legionella acquired from swimming pool water. The only possible case was in Japan where a 57-year-old male was admitted to hospital with a high fever, productive cough and dyspnea. Six days before admission he had had an episode of near drowning in a public bath. Chest X-ray showed wide-spread pneumonia and acute renal failure. He died of septic shock. Culture of material obtained from a lung abscess revealed *L. pneumophila* serogroup 6. In addition, rhabdomyolysis was pathologically confirmed after autopsy (Tokuda *et al.* 1997).

It has been suggested that the more likely potential risk of being infected with legionella in swimming pool environments lies with using the showers rather than the pool itself, particularly where the showers are poorly maintained. To reduce the risk shower water should be stored at 60 °C to reduce the growth of *Legionella* spp. (WHO 2005b). In Germany *L. pneumophila* has been proposed as a parameter for judging the quality of swimming pool water (Hasselbarth 1992). One issue that should be considered is that swimming pools are used by a variety of people of all ages and health including those who may be immunocompromised and thus more susceptible to infection from opportunist bacteria. Control measures are discussed in detail by Surman *et al.* (2005).

Occurrence or likely occurrence of legionella in hot tubs and saunas

Hot tubs (shallow pools containing warm water with air injection through holes in the bottom or the wall used for relaxation) and saunas, like hot springs, provide suitable environments for colonisation by *Legionella* spp. due to the warm temperatures of the environment. The majority of cases of Legionnaires' disease and Pontiac fever associated with recreational waters appear to be associated with hot tubs (Table 4.6). A number of studies from around the world have demonstrated the frequent presence of *Legionella* spp. in hot tubs even if there was no reported case of Legionnaires' disease. Groothuis *et al.* (1985) for example, took water samples from hot tubs in The Netherlands with water temperatures between 35 °C and 40 °C and free available chlorine less than 0.3 mg/l, and from 50 swimming pools. *L. pneumophila* was found in 11 out of 28 hot tubs tested and from two of the swimming pools investigated. The swimming pools had a lower temperature (between 8 °C and 38 °C) than the hot tubs, which was given as the explanation for the lower incidence of legionella.

Kuroki *et al.* (1998) surveyed hot tubs in 11 private houses, 8 public baths and 13 spas in Japan. Free living ameobae that are known to be the hosts of legionella bacteria were isolated from 75% of the water samples. Single *Legionella* spp, *L. pneumophila* with different serogroups were isolated in concentrations ranging from 10^1 to 10^4 cfu/100 ml.

Some investigations have isolated legionellae from sand filters within hot tub systems (Goldberg *et al.* 1989; Miller *et al.* 1993). This occurs where the concentrations of biocides for decontamination of the hot tub water are too low within filter systems where organic material is trapped. Once legionellae are introduced into the hot tub circulation, the warm temperature of the water and the organically rich environment within the filter provide an ideal environment for multiplication and survival of the bacteria. The filter then acts as a reservoir for infection through the release of bacteria into the hot tub with the production of contaminated aerosols.

During January 1998, a number of people were taken ill in a hotel in Wisconsin, United States. They had all been exposed to the hotel's hot tub and swimming pool. Serological evidence was found of acute infection with *L. micdadei* and the patients were diagnosed with Pontiac fever. High concentrations of heterotrophic bacteria were isolated from the hot tub. *L. micdadei* was recovered from the swimming pool filter and water from the hot tub after heat enrichment but not from pools and hot tub in nearby hotels. Endotoxin was also isolated in the highest concentrations in the water from the implicated hotel. From this study it is possible to conclude that endotoxin from legionellae or other bacteria may play a part in the pathogenesis of Pontiac fever (Fields *et al.* 2001).

Between June 24 and July 5, 1996, three patients were admitted to the same hospital in Japan with atypical pneumonia and elevated antibody titres for *L. pneumophila* serogroup 1. They had all visited the same hot tub prior to onset of the symptoms. *L. pneumophila* serogroup 1 was isolated from the hot tub's hot water tanks and outlets (Nakadate *et al.* 1999).

A 37-year-old woman in the United States was admitted to hospital with symptoms of a sore throat, fever, headache, myalgia and shortness of breath. It was noticed that she became ill after using a hot tub, which her two children had also used and who had also developed a self-limited illness. Water from the hot tub was tested positive for *L. pneumophila*. The patient eventually recovered after treatment (Tolentino *et al.* 1996).

In Sweden in April 1999, 20 cases of febrile disorder with headache, myalgia and chest pain consistent with Pontiac fever were reported to the Swedish Institute for Infectious Disease Control (SMI). All the patients had stayed in the same hotel which contained an area with a sauna, two hot tubs and shower facilities. As the guests from the hotel had come from all over the country the SMI informed all infectious disease clinics and Country Medical Offices throughout Sweden. A retrospective cohort study was undertaken to identify activities responsible for transmission of the disease. Water samples from the hot tubs and showers were collected and the water temperature measured. Environmental swabs of biofilm from showers were collected in guest rooms and relaxation areas. No *Legionella* spp. were detected from the environmental samples. In total 72 people had symptoms of illness during or within two days of staying at the hotel. There were no fatalities. Cases of Pontiac fever were restricted to people who visited the hot tub area during a three-day-period. The attack rate during this period was 71%. *L. micdadei* was confirmed serologically in 20 out of 30 tested patients. This was considered sufficient to conclude that *L. micdadei* was the causative agent of the outbreak (Gotz *et al.* 2001).

Cases of Legionnaires' disease associated with display hot tubs

The largest outbreaks of Legionnaires' disease have been linked to display hot tubs.

An outbreak of Legionnaires' disease was reported from a trade fair in Belgium in November 1999. Clinical symptoms appeared in 80 people and Legionnaires' disease was confirmed in 13 of these. Four people died. The outbreak was traced to hot tubs which were exhibited at the show (De Schrijver 2003).

In June 1999 it was confirmed that 188 people who visited a large flower show near Amsterdam, The Netherlands, had contracted Legionnaires' disease and 28 people had died. Legionnaires' disease was considered probable in a further 55 cases. Of the affected, 17 people with confirmed and four with probable Legionnaires' disease died. The public health laboratory found legionellae in a hot tub that was on display at the show. The strain of legionellae found in the hot tub was identical to that found in some of the patients (van Steenbergen *et al.* 1999).

In southwest Virginia, United States, in October 1996, Legionnaires' disease was confirmed in five people in neighbouring towns and a case-control study was undertaken to identify exposures associated with the illness. It was discovered that 93% of cases in the case-control study had visited a home-improvement store and 77% of these remembered walking past a display hot tub. An environmental investigation later confirmed the spa as the source of the infection. Sputum isolates from two cases were an exact match to the hot tub filter isolate from the store (Benkel *et al.* 2000).

In June 2000 a 32-year-old Australian woman was reported as being critically ill after contracting Legionnaires' disease. The disease was also confirmed in two men. All of the affected people were at the same football club and the source of infection was traced to the club's hot tub (source: http://www.hcinfo.com/outbreaks-news.htm).

A man died in the United Kingdom in Febraury 2001 after being exposed to a display hot tub at a garden centre in Bagshot, Surrey, United Kingdom. The man fell ill two days after visiting the garden centre and later died (Anonymous 2001a).

Travel-related Legionnaires' disease

Travel-related Legionnaires' disease presents particular issues since source identification is difficult. There is a significant gap between population-based estimates of the frequency of Legionnaires' disease and national surveillance data. This is worse for outbreaks of travel-related cases of the disease since travellers may become ill, often far from the source of infection, up to 14 days after exposure to legionellae, making clusters of cases difficult to detect (Jernigan *et al.* 1996). Travellers exposed to the infection towards the end of their travel would probably not develop symptoms until returning home, where an association with recent travel may be missed. Outbreaks of Legionnaires' disease are often detected by identifying community clusters of infections. Because people staying in a hotel or on a cruise ship are from various different countries or towns, the association with the hotel or ship may not be recognised. In addition, physicians often do not suspect or confirm the diagnosis of Legionnaires' disease in patients with community-acquired pneumonia.

Jernigan *et al.* (1996) report that in an unpublished review undertaken by the CDC between 1985 and 1993 about 23% of cases of Legionnaires' disease in the United States were associated with travel in the ten days before the onset of the disease. The figure is higher for Europe. CDSC report that at least 45% of cases in England and Wales are travel related (Joseph *et al.* 1993). Although these are not all linked to use of recreational waters, risk factors do include the use of hot springs and hot tubs (Grist *et al.* 1979; Joseph *et al.* 1994). There is likely to have been increased detection of Legionnaires' disease in Europe since the establishment of a computerised surveillance system based in England in 1986, linking 31 countries Europe-wide. The European Working Group for Legionella Infections supports a surveillance scheme for travel associated Legionnaires' disease, the standardisation of water sampling methods, legionella typing methods and the validation of diagnostic methods.

On July 14, 1994, it was reported that three persons had been admitted to hospital in New York, United States, with atypical pneumonia. All three had been passengers on the same cruise ship three weeks earlier. Another three cases were identified and it was confirmed that urine specimens from the first three cases were positive for *L. pneumophila* serogroup 1. A confirmed case of Legionnaires' disease was defined as physician-diagnosed pneumonia with laboratory evidence of legionella infection in a passenger or crew member who had travelled on the cruise ship between March 1 and July 20, 1994, with onset of illness occurring after the second day of the cruise and within 14 days after the end of the cruise. To determine the outbreak, cases of confirmed or probable Legionnaires' disease identified before July 31, 1994, were enrolled into a matched case-control study. Water and environmental swabs were collected from 28 sites on board the ship, sites visited by passengers in Bermuda and from the ship's source of water in New York, United States. The case-control study showed that case-passengers were significantly more likely than control-passengers to have been in the hot tub water. Among the passengers who did not enter the hot tub water, case passengers were significantly more likely to have spent time around the hot tub (Anonymous 1994).

The hot tubs seem to have been a persistent source of infection for at least nine separate week-long cruises during the spring and summer of 1994. No further cases of Legionnaires' disease were identified after the hot tubs were closed on July 16, 1994 (Jernigan *et al.* 1996).

IV Conclusions

The major concern regarding Legionnaires' disease and recreational use of water is associated with the use of, and proximity to, hot tubs, although there are a number of reported isolations of *Legionella* spp. from swimming pool showers and open waters.

The illness is considered to be severe with a high risk of death, severe acute symptoms generally lasting more than seven days. There are a number of documented cases of persons suffering sequelae as a consequence of infection.

Legionellosis	Epidemiological evidence linking recreational water use with illness	Evidence from outbreak data of illness associated with recreational water	Documented cases of illness associated with recreational water	Documented cases of sequelae (in any situation)
	√	√	√	√

LEPTOSPIRA

Credibility of association with recreational water: Strongly associated

I Organism

Pathogen

The aetiological agents of leptospirosis are the pathogenic bacteria, leptospires.

Taxonomy

The family Leptospiraceae are of the order Spirochaetales and are divided into three genera: *Leptospira, Leptonema* and *Turneria*. Taxonomy classifies *Leptospira* into 12 species: *L. alexanderi, L. biflexa, L. borgpetersenii, L. fainei, L. inadai, L. interrogans, L. kirschneri, L. noguchii, L. santarosai, L. weilii, L. meyeri,* and *L. wolbachii*. All recognised species have been classified as pathogens, intermediate or saprophytes (Plank and Dean 2000). The severe forms of disease are caused by serovars of *L. interrogans: australis, autumnalis, bataviae, copenhageni, icterohaemorrhagiae* (carried primarily by rats and often associated with water sports and immersion), *javanica* and *lari*. Although most leptospires are associated with mild illness, these serovars are frequently fatal if untreated.

Reservoir

The primary source of leptospires is the surface of the renal tubes in the kidney of an excreting carrier animal. Carrier animals pass urine containing leptospires into the surrounding environment.

Distribution

Worldwide. The highest prevalence rates are in tropical, developing countries although epidemiological studies show infection in temperate zones is more frequent than previously thought (Plank and Dean 2000).

Charactersitics

Pathogenic leptospires are aerobic, motile, helicoidal, flexible spirochaetes, usually between 6 μm and 20 μm long and 0.1 μm in diameter, with hooked ends.

II Health aspects

Primary disease symptoms and sequelae

Mild forms of leptospirosis (also known as Weil's disease or haemorrhagic jaundice) range from a febrile incapacitating illness lasting between 10 and 20 days, consisting of severe muscle pains, meningism and mild renal incapacity, to a barely detectable subclinical infection. Severe forms are frequently fatal if untreated; symptoms include jaundice, haemorrhage, potentially fatal kidney and liver failure. Aseptic meningitis is estimated to complicate between 5% and 24% of cases (Arean 1962; De Brito *et al.* 1979).

Sequelae include psychiatric illness such as depression and psychoses, prolonged listlessness and joint pains lasting from weeks to months. Shpilberg *et al.* (1990) evaluated 11 patients who had had acute leptospirosis for possible sequelae. Results showed that liver and renal disease had resolved but headache and ophthalmic sequelae persisted. Delirium, hallucinations, encephalitis, grand mal seizures and coma have been reported (Torre *et al.* 1994).

An association between antiphospholipid syndrome and leptospirosis has been proposed by Tattevin *et al.* (2003). The authors describe a case in a 63-year-old man who was admitted to hospital with fever, acute renal failure, lymphocytic meningitis, hepatitis, and alveolar meningitis. Leptospirosis was suspected and confirmed. However, the patient was also showing pulmonary hypertension which has not been reported in leptospirosis but is associated with antiphospholipid syndrome (Karmochkine *et al.* 1996; Levine *et al.* 2002). Once the patient was treated with amoxicillin the pulmonary hypertension resolved and kaolin clotting time, which was slower than normal in the patient, also returned to normal. Levels of antibodies to antiphospholipid returned to normal suggesting that antiphospholipid syndrome and leptospirosis were associated.

In a retrospective study of 16 patients with documented leptospirosis, IgG anticardiolipin antibody concentrations were increased in all patients with severe leptospirosis but in none of the patients with uncomplicated leptospirosis (Rugman *et al.* 1991). Tattevin *et al.* (2003) conclude that although antiphospholipid antibodies are found in patients with leptospirosis, they may be associated with more severe infection and with particular symptoms of antiphospholipid syndrome.

Erythroid hypoplasia has been found to be associated with leptospirosis but is rarely reported. Two literature reports are described (Nicodema *et al.* 1989; Somers *et al.* 2003). Thrombocytopenia in a patient with serological findings indicative of acute leptospira infection is reported by Wenz *et al.* (2001).

Disease manifestations are not necessarily due to direct tissue damage by the organism, but due to the host's immune response. Leptospira may persist in the brain – in one report 4 out of 11 patients had persistent headaches for between 6 and 34 years post-infection. Ophthalmic involvement with blurred vision has been reported to persist for decades following acute infection (Shpilberg *et al.* 1990).

Cardiac involvement is common in severe disease and can manifest as myocarditis, congestive heart failure, non-specific electrocardiogram abnormalities and sudden death. Uncommon sequelae are acalculous cholecystitis, pancreatitis, and hypermylasemia (Plank and Dean 2000). Acute respiratory failure necessitating mechanical ventilation may occur rarely. This may be caused by adult respiratory distress syndrome or profuse pulmonary bleeding. Two cases are described by de Koning *et al.* (1995) from The Netherlands. One person died and the other recovered completely.

Exposure/mechanism of infection

Leptospires enter the host from contaminated urine, water, soil or mud, by penetrating abrasions in the skin or body surfaces and possibly by inhalation of aerosols containing leptospires. It is thought that they do not penetrate the skin unless it is wet.

Disease incidence

The incidence of human infection is higher in the tropics than in temperate regions but transmission occurs in both industrialised and developing countries. Incidence rates are underestimated due to lack of awareness of the disease and relatively inaccessible and insufficiently rapid diagnostics (Bharti *et al.* 2003). Farr (1995) estimated that an average of between 100 and 200 cases are identified annually in the United States with about 50% of cases occurring in Hawaii.

Surveillance information is collected by the International Leptospirosis Society and reported in collaboration with the WHO. Data collected in 1999 concerning number of deaths and mortality rates are provided in Table 4.7.

Incubation period

Incubation varies from 5 to 14 days. Patients suffer a very sudden onset of severe headache, fever, muscle pain and sometimes red eyes and photophobia.

Infectivity

A very small number (one to ten) of leptospires can cause a fatal infection in a susceptible host. Leptospires enter a host from urine, water, soil or mud, by penetrating small abrasions in the skin or body surfaces, possibly by inhalation of aerosols containing leptospires, and possibly through the conjunctival sac. Drinking or inhalation of contaminated water following immersion has also caused leptospirosis. Once in the body the leptospires spread very quickly and can be found in the blood minutes after entering the body of the host. Between two and four weeks later leptospires appear in the kidney. They can enter the brain and the anterior chamber of the eye. Around 90% of recognised cases of leptospirosis are mild and self-limited (Plank and Dean 2000).

Table 4.7 Annual average number of deaths associated with leptospirosis globally (WHO 1999)

Country	Number of deaths in ten years	Annual number of deaths (average)	Mortality rate per 100,000 population
Australia	4	0.4	0.2
Barbados	73	7.3	23.6
Brazil	2502	250	0.8
Bulgaria	12.7	1.3	3
China:			
Beijing		579	7.9
Chengdu	1570	157	6.8
Fuzhou	68	6.8	1
Wuhan	848	84.8	2.1
Costa Rica	17	1.7	5.3
Guadaloupe	16	1.6	13.7
Hungary	11	1.1	3.5
India:			
Chennai	32	3.2	13.9
Kerala	52	5.2	3.7
Madras	32	3.2	13.9
Mumbai	30	3.0	17.6
Italy	161	16.1	12.6
Japan		5	15.2
The Netherlands	17	1.7	4.9
New Caladonia	40	4	2.6
Romania	114	11.4	0.38
Russian Federation	57.5	3.8	
Seychelles	60–80	7	9.3
Slovakia	1	0.1	0.2
Switzerland	3	0.3	5.3
Thailand	10	1	5
The United Kingdom	19	1.9	4.5
The United States	8	0.8	1.50

Sensitive groups

Leptospirosis used to be considered as an occupational disease, associated with activities such as mining, sewer maintenance, livestock farming, butchering, veterinary medicine, and military manoeuvres, particularly to tropical areas. The relative importance of such occupational risks has decreased since protective measures have been implemented. Many cases occur in association with conditions of slum living or with recreational activities involving immersion in water (Anonymous 1998; Haake *et al.* 2002). In tropical environments, occupational exposure such as rice farming and other agricultural activities is still significant, as well as exposure of the general population during activities of daily living, and especially is associated with high seasonal rainfall. Leptospirosis is the only epidemic-prone infection which can be transmitted directly from contaminated water. The occurrence of flooding after heavy rainfall facilitates the spread of the organism due to the proliferation of rodents which shed large amounts of leptosires in their urine (WHO 2005c). Of significance is the potential for large, multinational, point-source outbreaks after recreational events (Bharti *et al.* 2003).

III Evidence for association of leptospirosis with recreational waters

Leptospires can survive in water apparently indefinitely, depending on acidity. Farmers, sewer workers, miners, fishermen and meat workers have historically been at highest risk of infection. Recently, however, a number of outbreaks have been associated with recreational water contact – the majority associated with fresh open water accessible to animals; recreational exposure to natural water sources is reported as a common route of transmission (Jackson *et al.* 1993). In the United States, for example, prior to 1970 it was suggested that 66% of cases were from occupational exposure (Heath *et al.* 1965). In 1971, however, 60% of reported cases were in children, students, and housewives while only 17% occurred among occupational workers, suggesting the epidemiology had moved to home and recreational settings (Thiermann 1977).

Infection has occurred through activities such as wading (Trevejo *et al.* 1995), swimming and rafting, especially among travellers undertaking 'adventure tourism' in endemic countries (Levett 1999; Haake *et al.* 2002). Of 237 confirmed cases in The Netherlands between 1987 and 1991, 14% were diagnosed in travellers, all except one who had had surface water exposure overseas (Van Crevel *et al.* 1994).

In June and August 1964, in the State of Washington, United States, 61 cases of leptospirosis occurred in teenagers who reported swimming in a local irrigation canal. When the canal was inspected it was found that a herd of cattle had access to the water upstream of the swimming area. A number of these cattle were found to be carrying antibodies against *L. pamona*.

Anderson *et al.* (1978) report seven cases of leptospirosis in children aged between 11 and 16 years old in Tennessee, United States, during August 1975. Antibodies to *L. grippotyphosa* were found in all of them. All had a history of swimming in a local creek. Although no leptospires were found in water samples taken from the suspected area in which a herd of cows were present with access to the water, possibly indicating the source of infection.

In September 1987, 22 United States military personnel were infected with leptospires on the island of Okinawa, Japan. The source was considered to be the Aha Falls where the affected individuals had swum. Epidemiological investigation showed a significant association between those who had swallowed water and infection but just immersion in the water was not significantly associated with infection (Corwin *et al.* 1990).

Also in 1987, eight individuals were identified with symptoms of leptospirosis on the island of Kauai, Hawaii (Katz *et al.* 1991). All eight had been swimming in a local river. Six were shown to have infection by *L. australis*, one an infection of *L. bataviae* and one a *L. fort bragg* infection. A tenuous link was made to a herd of cattle in an adjacent field, eight of which were found with antibodies to *L. hardjo* and *L. bataviae*.

Jackson *et al.* (1993) report five cases of leptospirosis in boys from a town in Illinois, United States, who had been swimming in a particular area. Epidemiological investigations revealed that the boys had swallowed water whilst swimming, but this was the only risk factor identified. Cattle in the area were serologically positive for *L. grippotyphosa* and water samples showed positive for *L. grippotyphosa*.

In October 1996, it was reported that five patients from Illinois, United States, were suffering from an unknown febrile illness. They had returned from a white-water rafting trip in Costa Rica. Investigators interviewed all 26 participants on the trip to assess symptoms and potential environmental and behavioural risk factors. Risk for the illness was associated with having ingested river water and being submerged under water after falling into the river whilst rafting (Anonymous 1997).

In July 1998, CDC began investigating an outbreak of acute febrile illness among athletes from 44 states and seven countries who participated in triathlons in Illinois, United States, on June 21, 1998, and in Wisconsin, United States on July 5, 1998. A suspected case of leptospirosis was defined as onset of fever during June 21 and August 13, 1998 in a triathlon participant that was associated with at least two of the following symptoms: chills, headache, myalgia, diarrhoea, eye pain or red eyes. Of the 1194 athletes that participated in one or both events, 110 described an illness meeting the case definition (Anonymous 1998).

In September 2000, CDC was notified of at least 20 cases of acute febrile illness in three counties who had participated in a multisport expedition race in Borneo, Malaysia, during August and September. Of the 304 athletes who participated in the event 158 were contacted for details of symptoms. Of these, 83 reported chills, 80 headache, and 58 diarrhoea. Arthralgias was reported by 47 athletes, dark urine by 44, and calf/leg pain by 45. In total, 68 patients met the case definition. Epidemiological, serological and immunohistochemical staining evidence for leptospirosis was obtained from 32 athletes suggesting that leptospira was the etiologic agent causing disease. Significant exposure risks included kayaking, swimming in, and swallowing water from, the Segama River (Anonymous 2001b).

Two outbreaks have been associated with non-chlorinated swimming pools (Cockburne *et al.* 1954; de Lima *et al.* 1990).

Lee *et al.* (2002) report 21 cases of leptospirosis between 1999 and 2000 in Guam State, United States. The disease was contracted from a lake during an adventure race. Leptospira was confirmed by serology, and an epidemiologic investigation demonstrated that swimming in the reservoir, head submersion in the water and swallowing water while swimming were risk factors for illness. Water samples were not tested and an environmental assessment of the reservoir was not conducted.

Somers *et al.* (2003) report a case of erythroid hypoplasia in a 30-year-old man admitted to hospital in Dublin, Ireland, with Weil's disease. He had a recent history of canoeing in the river Liffey in Dublin. The man was experiencing erythroid hypoplasia (anaemia, reticulocytopenia and bone marrow erythropcytopenia) in association with leptospiral infection.

Surveillance data

The data in Table 4.8 are derived from the history of cases and bathing in small ponds and rivers in Slovakia. Most of the cases were attributed to *L. grippotyhosa* and *L. icterohaemorrh*.

Between 1990 and 1996, 55 cases out of 252 (22%) of leptospirosis in England and Wales were documented as being related to recreational activities such as windsurfing, swimming, scuba diving and fishing (Hartigan 1982). Other recreational activities include water-skiing and golfing (Grennan 1996).

Between 1994 and 1996 there were 222 reports of leptospirosis made to the Italian Ministry of Health. In comparison with the preceding eight-year-period, the risk of contracting leptospirosis from recreational activities was found to have increased from 34.7% to 38.2% (Cacciapuoti *et al.* 1994). All cases except two were thought to have been contracted in Italy. Of the 103 cases for whom information on risk factors was available, 95.1% were patients at risk for one or more of the following factors: place of residence, contact with animals, occupational and recreational activities. Of the 55 cases for which the mode of transmission was known, 38% were ascribed to recreational activities – this includes fishing (six cases), bathing (three cases) and canoeing (three cases). In Italy, as well as in many other countries, the disease is thought to be under-reported, in particular, the febrile forms of the disease (Ciceroni *et al.* 2000).

Table 4.8 Cases of leptospirosis 1987–1998 in Slovakia (Source: M. Spalekova, personal communication).

Year	Total number of cases	Incidence per 100 000	Cases exposed to water
1987	36	0.7	15
1988	67	1.3	43
1989	72	1.4	40
1990	30	0.6	5
1991	33	0.6	0
1992	34	0.6	4
1993	29	0.5	3
1994	37	0.7	4
1995	33	0.6	24
1996	25	0.5	0
1997	39	0.7	5
1998	26	0.5	1

IV Conclusions

There is clear epidemiological evidence and outbreak data linking cases of leptospirosis to persons using water for recreational purposes. However, *Leptospira* spp. are usually associated with animals that urinate into surface waters, and swimming-associated outbreaks attributed to *Leptospira* are rare. Human leptospirosis is primarily a problem in tropical countries but has also appeared as a sporadic health issue in Europe, Japan, Australia and the United States. The acute illness is considered moderately severe but is often prolonged. There is a moderate probability of developing long-term sequelae.

Leptospirosis	Epidemiological evidence linking recreational water use with illness	Evidence from outbreak data of illness associated with recreational water	Documented cases of illness associated with recreational water	Documented cases of sequelae (in any situation)
	√	√	√	√

MYCOBACTERIUM

Credibility of association with recreational water: Strongly associated

I Organism

Pathogen

Mycobacterium.

Taxonomy

Mycobacterium is the only genus in the family Mycobacteriaceae, order Actinomycetales. Over 70 species have been defined, of which at least 30 cause disease in humans and animals. There are about 16 species that have been associated with water. The most significant of the environmental mycobacteria in terms of public health is the *Mycobacterium avium* complex (MAC), which includes *M. avium*, and *M. intracellulare* (WHO 2004c). Table 4.9 shows the non-tuberculous mycobacteria with pathogenic potential frequently found in environmental habitats.

Table 4.9 Non tuberculous mycobacterium that cause infection in immunocompromised and immunocompetent hosts (Adapted from Collier *et al.* 1998)

Non-tuberculous mycobacterium that cause infection in immunocompetent hosts	Non-tuberculous mycobacterium that cause infection in AIDS patients	Non-tuberculous mycobacterium that cause infection in immunocompromised hosts (not AIDS patients)
MAC *	MAC*	MAC*
M. kansaii *	*M. kansaii* *	*M. fortuitum complex* *
M. marinum *	*M. genavense*	*M. kansaii* *
M. fortuitum complex *	*M. haemophilum*	*M. xenopi* *
M. xenopi *	*M. malmoense* *	*M. haemophilum*
M. simiae *	*M. xenopi* *	*M. marinum* *
M. szulgai	*M. szulgai*	*M. scrofulaceum*
M. malmoense *	*M. simiae* *	
M. ulcerans *	*M. celatum*	
M. smegmatis *	*M. marinum* *	
M. haemophilum		
M. scrofulaceum		
M. shirmoidei		
M. asiaticum		

*associated with water

The majority of non-tuberculous mycobacterium respiratory isolates are MAC but only about half of these are pathogenic (O'Brien *et al.* 1987).

Reservoir

Mycobacterium has been recovered in almost every environment that is in contact with susceptible species including humans, animals, birds and fish, including surface waters.

Distribution

Worldwide, including north America, Europe, Asia, Africa and Australia (von Reyn *et al.* 1993). Since it is not a micro-organism that is analysed for routinely in water samples its presence may be underestimated.

Characteristics

M. avium is a member of the "slow-growing mycobacteria". This is a consequence of the presence of a single rRNA gene cluster (Bercovier *et al.* 1986), long chain fatty acids, and the impermeable cell wall (Brennan and Nikaido 1995). *M. avium* can grow at 45°C and at reduced oxygen levels (Mijs *et al.* 2002). Highest growth range occurs within the pH range 5–6 (George and Falkinham 1986). These characteristics result in the resistance of *M. avium* to antibiotics (Rastogi *et al.* 1981), heavy metals (Miyamoto *et al.* 2000) and disinfectants (Taylor *et al.* 2000).

II Health aspects

Primary disease symptoms and sequelae

Infection by MAC produces symptoms including cough, sputum production, fatigue, weight loss, sweats, haemoptysis, pleuritic and non-pleuritic chest pain. Failure to diagnose and treat the disease may result in lung damage. In those patients who have no previous lung damage, symptoms include fever, fatigue, sweats, weight loss, dyspnea, haemoptysis and chest pain. Malabsorption is a common but not universal result of intestinal MAC infection (Gray and Rabeneck 1989).

The severity of mycobacterial diseases varies. High morbidity and mortality is associated with disseminated infections of *M. avium* in AIDS patients (Horsburgh *et al.* 1994; 2001). In non-HIV/AIDS patients the severity ranges from relatively mild cases of hypersensitivity pneumonitis to life threatening respiratory infections in people with underlying lung pathology or immunological defects and occasionally in those with no known predisposing conditions. *M. avium* sub species *M. paratuberculosis* is suspected to be associated with Crohn's disease (Herman-Taylor *et al.* 1998; Fouad *et al.* 2001; Herman-Taylor 2001).

Pickles *et al.* (2001) report a case of a 48-year-old man who was suffering general malaise, a productive cough, weight loss and non-specific aches over a period of two months. Following a caecal biopsy it was suspected that he was infected with mycobacteria enterocolites or systematic *M. avium intracellulare*. He started antimycobacterial therapy which was continued for one year. The man was found to have occasional granulomas which was confirmed as Crohn's disease. The relationship between *M. avium intracellulare* and Crohn's disease is not fully understood, although there is a growing body of evidence to support *M. avium intracellulare* as a causative factor in the development of Crohn's disease. For now Crohn's disease should be regarded as a disorder resulting from a combination of genetic and environmental factors (Pickles *et al.* 2001).

Hypersensitivity pneumonitis is seen in immunocompetent persons with aerosol exposure to mycobacteria and is typically linked to hot tubs and indoor swimming pools. Lifeguards and other persons working in such environments are particularly thought to be at risk (Embil *et al.* 1997; Mangione *et al.* 2001; Mery and Horan 2002). The organisms are found in higher densities in the air above indoor pools than in the pool water itself. Due to their hydrophobic nature they can be found adhering to surfaces. Following inhalation symptoms include cough, dyspnea, fatigue, impaired exercise tolerance and sputum production. Discontinuation of exposure leads to an improvement of the symptoms (Rickman *et al.* 2002).

Treatment includes a course of antibiotics for many months. Patients with pre-existing lung disease may require surgery although there is a risk of complications such as bronchopleural fistulas (Iseman *et al.* 1985; Shiraishi *et al.* 2002). Surgery is generally only necessary where patients have failed medical treatment or for severe symptomatic disease. When present, localised disease is treated with surgical intervention. Surgery is associated with relatively high morbidity and there are a number of cases described in the literature (Shiraishi *et al.* 2002).

MAC is a rare cause of osteomyelitis (Chan *et al.* 2001). Whitehead *et al.* (2003) report a case of a 61-year-old man who developed septic arthritis of an interphalangeal joint and osteomyelitis of the phalanx due to *M. malmoense*. The man was immunocompromised, already suffering from rheumatoid arthritis and had a history of poor healing of skin lesions, suggesting a reduced immune response. The environment, e.g. water, has been suggested as the principal source of infection for *M. malmoense*. In Sweden, 221 cases have been described over a 22-year-period and was second to *M. avium* as a cause of atypical mycobacterial infection. In the United Kingdom it is the second most common cause of non-tuberculous lymphadenitis (Pozniak and Bull 1999).

Table 4.10 Cases of disease caused by mycobacteria in recreational waters

Species	Disease	Source/ setting	Affected	Reference
MAC	Pulmonary disease	Hot tub	Family of five	Mangione *et al.* 2001
MAC	Pulmonary disease	Hot tub	Family of five	Embil *et al.* 1997
MAC	Cutaneous infection	Circulating bath water	Three people	Sugita *et al.* 2000
MAC	Hypersensitivity pneumonitis	Hot tub	Two case studies	Rickman *et al.* 2002
M. fortuitum	Furunculosis	Footbaths at a nail salon	110 people	Winthrop *et al.* 2002
M. absessus	Sporotrichoid dermatosis	Public bath	Two case studies	Lee *et al.* 2000b
M. kansaii	Cellulitis	Swimming at a beach	One immuno-compromised patient	Hsu *et al.* 2002

IV Conclusions

There is clear evidence for the association of MAC with recreational waters. The species of Mycobacterium that are associated with water are associated with a variety of diseases. Some, such as *M. ulverans* are pathogenic in previously healthy individuals, others, such as *M. avium*, usually cause disease in compromised individuals. The majority of cases associated with recreational waters appear to be attributed to swimming pools and hot tubs resulting in skin and soft tissue infections in immunocompetent patients. However, hypersensitivity pneumonitis is also seen in immunocompetent persons with aerosol exposure to mycobacteria. Lifeguards and other persons working in such environments are particularly thought to be at risk.

Mycobacterium	Epidemiological evidence linking recreational water use with illness	Evidence from outbreak data of illness associated with recreational water	Documented cases of illness associated with recreational water	Documented cases of sequelae (in any situation)
	√	√	√	√

SALMONELLA

Credibility of association with recreational water: Strongly associated

I Organism

Pathogen

Bacteria from the genus *Salmonella*.

Taxonomy

The genus *Salmonella* is a member of the family Enterobacteriaceae. Members of the genus *Salmonella* are grouped according to their somatic (O) and flagellar (H) antigens. The genus has been divided into more than 2000 species on the basis of the differences in their cell wall (Popoff *et al.* 2000). With regards to enteric illness, *Salmonella* spp. can be divided into two groups: the typhoidal species (*S. typhi* and *S. paratyphi*) and the non-typhoidal species.

Reservoir

Salmonella bacteria live in the intestinal tracts of humans and other animals, including birds and reptiles. All salmonellae except for *S. typhi* and *S. paratyphi* are found in animals as well as humans. Excretion by humans and animals of potential pathogenic micro-organisms in their faeces may result in contamination of receiving waters (Ashbolt 1996).

Distribution

Distribution is worldwide. In many less developed regions of the world, where most typhoid fever cases occur, surveillance and outbreak investigation are limited by a lack of laboratory facilities; consequently there are no accurate data on the frequency or extent of typhoid fever worldwide.

Over the past three decades, practically all countries in Europe have reported a sharp rise in salmonellosis incidence (including foodborne outbreaks). The same pattern could be observed in a number of countries in the Eastern Mediterranean Region and south-east Asia Region (WHO 1997). Conflicting reports come from the Republic of Korea where a decrease in incidence has been reported since the 1970s (Yoo *et al.* 2002).

There was a ten-fold increase in the number of human cases of multi-drug resistant *S. typhimurium* DT 104 in the six-year-period between 1990 and 1996 rising from 300 to 3500 cases per year in the United Kingdom (England and Wales). This specific strain was second only to *S. enteriditis* as the most common salmonella in humans in the United Kingdom (England and Wales) in 1995 and more than 55% of cases of *S. typhimurium* in humans were caused by the multi-drug resistant DT 104. Infection with multi-drug resistant *S. typhimurium* DT 104 has been associated with hospitalisation rates which are twice that of other zoonotic foodborne salmonella infections and with ten times higher case-fatality rates.

An increase in overall number and percentage of multi-drug resistant *S. typhimurium* DT 104 is also reported from other European countries. In Germany, it accounted for up to 10% in more than 10,000 salmonella samples from human sources examined in 1995, and 18% of those examined in 1996. Almost all DT 104 isolates were multi-drug resistant with the same resistance pattern as in the United Kingdom (England and Wales). *S. typhimurium* DT 104 was detected in the United States in the late 1990s and may have spread widely in the United States.

Characteristics

Salmonella bacteria are rod shaped with widths of between 0.7 μm and 1.5 μm and length between 2.0 μm and 5.0 μm. Salmonella bacteria can survive in moist environments and in the frozen state for several months. The bacteria can be distinguished by phenotypic and genetic properties – they are Gram-negative, and facultatively anaerobic and motile. Salmonella bacteria do not ferment lactose, but most form H_2S or gas from carbohydrate fermentation (Holt *et al.* 1994).

II Health aspects

Primary disease symptoms and sequelae

Salmonella bacteria cause a range of illnesses which range from asymptomatic to symptomatic infections. Most infections are brief, self-limited and mild. Of particular interest to this review is the more serious illnesses of typhoid and paratyphoid (enteric) fever. Typhoid fever is caused by infection due to *S. typhi*; paratyphoid fever is due to infection with *S. paratyphi*.

S. *typhi* and *S. paratyphi* A, unlike most other *Salmonella* species, are harboured by humans and not animals, although livestock can occasionally be a source of *S. paratyphi* (WHO 2004a). Most other salmonellae primarily infect animals. Transmission is via faecally contaminated food and water. Non-typhoidal salmonellae infrequently cause waterborne outbreaks.

Four clinical types of salmonella infection may be distinguished: Gastroenteritis (ranging from mild to fulminant diarrhoea, nausea and vomiting); bacteraemia or septicaemia (high spiking fever with positive blood cultures); enteric fever (severe fever and diarrhoea) and lastly, a carrier state in persons with previous infections.

Acute systemic disease caused by *S. paratyphi* A and B, and *S. typhi* can invade tissues and cause septicaemia. Patients suffer from high temperatures rather than diarrhoea (WHO 1996). The illness caused by *S. typhi* is known as typhoid fever, common symptoms being headache, central nervous signs, malaise, anorexia, splenomegaly, and rose spots on the trunk (Hunter 1998).

Persons with diarrhoea usually recover completely, although it may be several months before their bowel habits are entirely normal. A small number of persons who are infected with salmonella, will go on to develop pains in their joints, irritation of the eyes, and painful urination. This is called Reiter's syndrome. It can last for months or years, and can lead to chronic arthritis which is difficult to treat and may cause long-term disabilities (Delcambre *et al.* 1983; Johnsen *et al.* 1983; Barth and Segal 1999). Antibiotic treatment does not make a difference to whether or not the person later develops arthritis. There are an estimated 500-plus fatal cases of salmonella each year in the United States; 2% of cases are complicated by chronic arthritis (http://www.cdc.gov.uk).

Complications of enteric fever include perforation of the bowel which occurs in between 0.5% and 5% of cases of typhoid (van Basten and Stockenbrugger 1994). Haemorrhage from bowel ulceration may occur early in the disease but as the disease progresses larger vessels may be involved. Continual faecal excretion of *S. typhi* is common for up to three months after infection but this may continue for up to a year. Evidence suggests that long-term carriers have an increased risk of hepatobiliary cancer which may be due to the production of N-nitroso compounds by the bacteria (Caygill *et al.* 1995).

S. typhi is often shed in the urine in the early stages of the disease and transient renal impairment is common (Khosla and Lochan 1991). The salmonellas of enteric fever may reside in many sites and may occur later as pyogenic lesions. Declercq *et al.* (1994) report abscesses in cancerous bone, brain and breast tissue. A case of pericardial abscess caused by *S. paratyphi* B in a patient in Malaysia has been described by Ahmed *et al.* (2001).

Most persons infected with non-typhoidal salmonella bacteria develop diarrhoea, fever, and abdominal cramps three to five days after infection. The illness is usually self-limiting lasting four to seven days after ingestion of contaminated food or water. However, salmonella infections are included in this review because in some persons the diarrhoea may be so severe that the patient needs to be hospitalised. In these patients the infection may spread from the intestines to the blood stream to cause septicaemia, consequently many organs become seeded with salmonella bacteria, sometimes leading to osteomyelitis, pneumonia or meningitis (Volk *et al.* 1991).

Exposure/mechanism of infection

Infection is primarily through the faecal–oral route, either from animal-to-animal or animal-to-human. Human-to-human transmission can occur where close contact is common, for example in special care units or residential homes (WHO 1997).

Diarrhoea is produced as a result of invasion by the salmonellae bacteria of the epithelial cells in the terminal portion of the small intestine. The bacteria then migrate to the lamina propria layer of the ileocaecal region, where their multiplication stimulates an inflammatory response which both confines the infection to the gastro intestinal tract and mediates the release of prostaglandins. These in turn activate cyclic adenosine monophosphate and fluid secretion, resulting in diarrhoea. *Salmonella* bacteria do not appear to produce enterotoxins. The severity of disease depends on the serotype of the organism, the number of bacteria ingested and the host susceptibility.

Disease incidence

Reported incidence and mortality associated with typhoid varies between geographical regions. Although there are indications of an overall downward trend in the global incidence of typhoid (e.g. in Thailand, Chile and Peru), certain regions continue to have high disease burdens (e.g. Indonesia and Viet Nam) (Hoffman *et al.* 1984) and large outbreaks have occurred (e.g. Tajikistan between 1996 and 1997 some 50,000 to 60,000 cases were reported annually; Pang *et al.* 1998).

At present it is not known whether these geographical differences are due to genetic variation in the local *S. typhi* strains, differences in the genetic susceptibility of host populations, or other factors such as the availability and use of vaccines. In 2003 WHO estimated the annual occurrence of typhoid fever at 16 million cases, with approximately 600,000 deaths worldwide (WHO 2003). Other figures estimate 21 million cases of typhoid fever and 200,000 deaths occur worldwide annually (Anonymous 2003).

An estimated 1.4 million cases of salmonellosis occur annually in the United States; of these, approximately 40,000 are culture-confirmed cases reported to CDC. There are approximately 1000 fatalities annually in the United States (http://www.cdc.gov). Approximately 30,000 cases are reported each year in the United Kingdom (Anonymous 1999). The majority of cases found in the literature were associated with food. Because many milder cases are not diagnosed or reported, the actual number of infections may be 20 or more times greater. Salmonellosis is more common in the summer than winter.

There are around 400 cases of typhoid fever per year in the United States, mostly among travellers (Anonymous 2003).

Incubation period

Varies from 1 to 14 days, average 3 to 5 days for typhoid fever (WHO 2004a).

Infectivity

Evidence shows that the infective dose for non-typhoidal salmonellosis is low. Hunter (1998) quotes below 1000 and possibly below ten organisms. Infective dose for *S. typhi* has been quoted by the Public Health Agency of Canada as 10,000 organisms (Health Canada 2001).

Sensitive groups

Children below the age of five years, the elderly and those with compromised immune systems are more likely to develop serious complications (Anonymous 2003) but typhoid fever affects all age groups. Species of *Salmonella* that normally cause diarrhoea (*S. enteritidis*, *S. cholera suis*) may become invasive in patients with particular predispositions such as cancer/sickle cell anaemia.

III Evidence for association of salmonellosis with recreational waters

The majority of cases of salmonellosis reported in the literature are associated with food. However, a number of studies from throughout the world have investigated the incidence and survival of salmonella in rivers, lakes, coastal water and beach sediments (Medema *et al.* 1995; Johnson *et al.* 1997; Polo *et al.* 1998). In these environments some, but not all, strains of salmonella are pathogenic, for reasons that are not clear (Kingsley *et al.* 2000). *S. typhi* does not survive well in polluted or warm waters but survival is extended in sediments (Holden 1970).

Storm water is often the major cause of water quality deterioration in receiving waters, especially at bathing areas. Storm water run-off may wash out fertilisers and food stuffs which, if prepared from animal products may be highly contaminated with salmonella bacteria (WHO 1996). In addition, seagulls have been shown to contribute salmonella in their faecal droppings to overnight roosting sites on lakes, open reservoirs and coastal waters (Fenlon 1981; Levesque *et al.* 1993; Geldreich 1996). Salmonella bacteria have frequently been isolated from receiving waters following wet weather events (Galès and Baluex 1992; Ferguson *et al.* 1996; Polo *et al.* 1998) presenting a risk to users.

Since 1995 only one outbreak of salmonellosis has been recorded by CDC from recreational waters in the United States. This was in March 1995, in Idaho. Three cases were recorded, the source being a swimming pool. The etiologic agent was identified as *S. java* (Levy *et al.* 1998).

According to Dufour (1984) the decrease in recorded outbreaks of enteric fever is partly due to the increase in sewage treatment plants using disinfection, especially in large population centres. Most outbreaks of enteric fever following swimming in fresh or marine water have usually involved grossly contaminated water (Parker 1990). The improvement of sanitation systems in developing countries will probably help to reduce the incidence of recreational waterborne outbreaks.

A number of cases of typhoid fever associated with drinking water were found in the published literature but only one described an association with recreational waters (PHLS 1959). Communication with the Statens Serum Institut, Copenhagen, Denmark, revealed five cases of salmonellosis associated with swimming pools between 1991 and 1994. Of these, three cases were imported from persons travelling to either Spain or Greece and two were in persons using paddling pools in Denmark. Three cases were attributed to *S. enteritidis*, one to *S. typhimurium* and one to *S. saint-paul* (Gunhild Hoy Kock-Hansen, personal communication).

IV Conclusions

Most persons infected with non-typhoidal salmonella bacteria develop diarrhoea, fever, and abdominal cramps which are usually self-limiting. However, typhoid fever is considered a severe disease, with hospitalisation and death occurring in many affected individuals. The probability of developing sequelae following infection with *S. typhi* and *S. paratyphi* is also high. The number of cases associated with recreational waters is low.

Typhoid fever	Epidemiological evidence linking recreational water use with illness	Evidence from outbreak data of illness associated with recreational water	Documented cases of illness associated with recreational water	Documented cases of sequelae (in any situation)
	√	√	√	√

SHIGELLA

Credibility of association with recreational waters: Strongly associated

I Organism

Pathogen

Bacteria from the genus *Shigella.*

Taxonomy

Shigella belong to the Family Enterobacteriaceae. The genus consists of four species: *S. dysenteriae* (type 1 produces the Shiga toxin), *S. flexneri*, *S. boydii*, and *S. sonnei* (mildest form).

Reservoir

Man and gorillas appear to be the only natural hosts for the shigellae (Nizeyi *et al.* 2001), where they remain localised in the intestinal epithelial cells.

Distribution

The bacteria are distributed worldwide.

Characteristics

Shigella is a gram-negative bacterium. The pathogenesis of the bacterium is based on it's ability to invade and replicate within the colonic epithelium, which results in severe inflammation and epithelial destruction (Jennison and Verma 2004). *Shigella* can be distinguished from other bacteria by phenotypic and genetic differences. They are facultatively anaerobic, non-spore-forming, non-motile bacilli which are serologically related to *E. coli. Shigella* are serotyped according to their somatic O antigens. Both group and type antigens are distinguished, group antigenic determinants being common to a number of related types.

II Health aspects

Primary disease symptoms and sequelae

Shigella bacteria cause bacillary dysentery (shigellosis). Shigellosis is primarily a paediatric disease. Symptoms can be mild or severe, depending on the species causing infection. Watery or bloody diarrhoea, abdominal pain, fever, and malaise are caused by *S. dysenteriae* type 1. Abdominal cramps, fever and watery diarrhoea occur early in the disease. Dysentery occurs during the ulceration process, with high concentrations of neutrofils in the stools.

The disease is generally self-limiting but has been included in this review because mortality is a possibility, particularly in malnourished children and in the elderly. The clinical illness is more likely to require hospitalisation than most other forms of infectious diarrhoea. If left untreated the clinical illness generally lasts between one day and one month with an average of seven days.

When associated with severe malnutrition it may precipitate complications. Reiter's syndrome is a late complication of *S. flexneri* infection, especially in persons with the genetic marker HLA-B27 (van Bohemen *et al.* 1986). HUS can occur after *S. dysenteriae* type 1 infection (Goldwater and Bettelheim 1995). Convulsions may occur in children; the mechanism may be related to a rapid rate of temperature elevation or metabolic alterations.

In some rare cases, *S. flexneri* infection may be associated with fulminating encephalopathy. Dieu-Osika *et al.* (1996) report the case of a six-year-old girl who was admitted to hospital with fever, diarrhoea and consciousness abnormalities in France. Brain CT scan was normal. *S. flexneri* type 2 was isolated from the stools. Despite antibiotic therapy, the encephalopathy was lethal. Two siblings were also infected, the first with only diarrhoea, the second with headache and mild consciousness abnormalities; both children recovered. The authors conclude that *S. flexneri* encephalopathy is associated with high mortality rate in developed countries.

Exposure/mechanism of infection

Shigella bacteria are transferred from person-to-person by contaminated water and food. With few exceptions the shigellae are harboured by humans and transferred easily by the faecal–oral route. Epidemics of shigellosis occur in crowded communities where human carriers exist.

Shigella spp. attach to, and invade the mucosal epithelium of the distal ileum and colon, causing inflammation and ulceration. However they rarely invade through the gut wall to the bloodstream. Enterotoxin is produced but its role in pathogenesis is uncertain since toxin negative mutants still produce disease.

In tropical countries direct person-to-person contact is probably the predominant route of transmission although food and waterborne spread are common. In developing countries, shigellosis is a common infection because of inadequate sewage disposal and lack of effectively treated water supplies. It is a cause of severe, potentially fatal, infection in children. Infection with shigella bacteria is of major importance in refugee camps or following natural disasters, when once again disposal of human faeces and the provision of clean water may be extremely difficult. It has been suggested that in some circumstances flies may spread the infection from person-to-person, as the disease is commonest at the time of year when the fly population is highest.

Disease incidence

Approximately 14,000 laboratory-confirmed cases of shigellosis and an estimated 448,240 total cases (mostly due to *S. sonnei*) occur in the United States each year. Because many milder cases are not diagnosed or reported, the actual number of infections may be 20 times greater (Anonymous 2003c).

In the developing world, *S. flexneri* predominates. Epidemics of *S. dysenteriae* type 1 have occurred in Africa and Central America with case-fatality rates of between 5% and 15% (WHO 2005d).

Shigella dysentries are responsible for about 60% of all cases of acute diarrhoea in children in Indonesia and India for example (Edmundson and Edmundson 1989). Dysentery has historically been regarded as a winter disease in Britain but the seasonal variation is now less well-marked (Newman 1993).

S. sonnei is the most common species of shigella in the United Kingdom and accounts for 90% of the isolates reported to the CDSC, United Kingdom. There were 695 laboratory reports of *S. sonnei* infection with all phage types in the United Kingdom (England and Wales) in 2000, compared with 907 in 1999 and 878 in 1998. In 1998 and 1999 the incidence was significantly higher in females than males and the age specific rate was highest in children aged one to four years and adults aged 25 to 29 years (CDSC 2000b).

Shigellosis causes 1.1 million deaths (WHO 2005d) and over 164 million cases each year, with the majority of cases occurring in the children of developing nations (Jennison and Verma 2004).

Incubation period

The incubation period for shigellosis varies from one to three days, with an average of 24 hours (Newman *et al.* 1993).

Infectivity

A small inoculum of *S. sonneri* or *S. flexneri* (up to 100 organisms) is sufficient to cause infection (Jennison and Verma 2004). As few as 10 *S. dysenteriae* bacilli can cause clinical disease.

Sensitive groups

In industrialised countries groups at increased risk of shigellosis include children in child-care centers, contacts of children in child-care settings, and persons in custodial institutions, where personal hygiene is difficult to maintain. In the United States Native Americans, orthodox Jews, international travellers, homosexual men and those in homes with inadequate water supplies for hand washing have been identified as vulnerable groups (Anonymous 2003c).

III Evidence for association of shigellosis with recreational waters

Though infection with shigella bacteria is not often spread by waterborne transmission, major outbreaks resulting from such transmission have been described.

A limited number of cases of shigellosis associated with recreational waters were found in the literature. Nevertheless some do exist with epidemiological evidence of association. In 1974 an outbreak of shigellosis associated with recreational water contact occurred among people using the Mississippi River (Rosenberg *et al.* 1976). A case-control study found a significant association with swimming. Among swimmers a significant association was found between the illness and getting water in the mouth. *S. sonnei* was isolated from the water.

Makintubee *et al.* (1987) report an outbreak of gastroenteritis due to *S. sonnei* in Oklahoma, United States during June 1982, which was traced to a single lake. A case-control study found that 14 of the 17 cases had visited the lake compared with three of the 17 controls. In a cohort study of 85 people who had visited the lake the risk of disease increased with exposure to lake water. Of those who were ill, 17% had waded in the lake, 20% had put their heads under water but had no water in their mouths and 62% had water in their mouths.

An artificial lake in Los Angeles, United States was suggested as the source of an outbreak of diarrhoea in 68 people in 1985. *S. sonnei* was isolated from 29 cases and *S. boydii* from four. Swallowing water, but not immersing the head without swallowing, and age under 15 years, were both found to be significantly associated with the disease (Sorvillo *et al.* 1988).

In 1989, an outbreak of shigellosis occurred among visitors to a recreational park in Michigan, United States. It was estimated that 65 cases of shigellosis were linked to swimming in a pond in the park. Shigella bacteria was not recovered from the pond. It was assumed that the swimmers themselves were the source (Blostein 1991).

In 1991 a group of people who had swum in Lake Oregon, United States suffered an outbreak of bloody diarrhoea. *S. sonnei* was identified as the cause in 38 cases. In a case-control study the most significant fact was swimming in the lake (P<0.001). Among swimmers, illness was associated with swallowing lake water (P<0.002) (Keene *et al.* 1994).

Surveillance data

Table 4.11 shows the number of cases of shigellosis associated with recreational waters in the United States between the years 1991 and 2000.

Table 4.11 Number of cases of shigellosis associated with recreational waters in the United States, 1991–2000 (Minnesota Department of Health 1974; Anonymous 1993; 1995; 1996b; Levy *et al.* 1998; Barwick *et al.* 2000; Lee 2002).

State	Date	Etiologic agent	Illness	No. cases	Source and setting
Rhode Island	July 1991	S. sonnei	GI	23	Lake, Swimming area
Mass.	June 1991	S. sonnei	GI	203	Lake, park
Virginia	July 1992	S. sonnei	GI	9	Lake, camp
New Jersey	June 1992	S. sonnei	GI	54	Lake, campground
Ohio	July 1993	S. sonnei	GI	150	Lake, park
New Jersey	June 1994	S. sonnei	GI	242	Lake, park
Minnesota	May 1994	S. flexneri	GI	35	Lake, park
Colorado	July 1995	S. sonnei	GI	81	Lake, recreational area
Colorado	July 1995	S. sonnei	GI	39	Lake, recreational area
Penn.	Aug. 1995	S. sonnei	GI	70	Lake, beach
Mass.	July 1997	S. sonnei	GI	9	Pool/ fountain, public park
Florida	1999	S. sonnei	GI	38	Interactive fountain, beach park
Missouri	Sept. 2000	S. flexneri	GI	6	Wading pool, municipal pool
Minnesota	July 2000	S. sonnei	GI	15	Lake/pond, beach
Minnesota	Aug. 2000	S. sonnei	GI	25	Lake, public beach

GI, gastroenteritis; Mass., Massachusetts; Penn., Pennsylvania

IV Conclusions

Epidemiological evidence exists for the association of recreational use of water and infection with shigella bacteria. All the cases reported were due to *S. sonnei* or *S. flexneri* which generally cause self-limiting illness. The species responsible for the more severe illness, *S. dysenteriae,* is more common in tropical regions but no cases associated with recreational waters were found in the literature. However, it is biologically plausible that *S. dysenteriae* could be encountered in freshwaters used for recreation.

Shigellosis	Epidemiological evidence linking recreational water use with illness	Evidence from outbreak data of illness associated with recreational water	Documented cases of illness associated with recreational water	Documented cases of sequelae (in any situation)
	√	√	√	√

VIBRIO VULNIFICUS

Credibility of association with recreational water: Strongly associated

I Organism

Pathogen
Vibrio vulnificus.

Taxonomy
V. vulnificus belongs to the Family Vibrionaceae, genus *Vibrio*.

Reservoir
V. vulnificus is a naturally occurring, free-living bacterium found in estuarine and marine environments.

Distribution
The organism is disributed worldwide. The bacteria are free-living inhabitants of estuarine and marine environments. They prefer tropical and subtropical climates where water temperatures are more than 18 °C. *V. vulnificus* prefers waters with low to moderate salinities (Motes *et al.* 1998; Strom and Paranjpye 2000).

Characteristics
V. vulnificus is a motile, Gram-negative, curved rod-shaped bacterium with a single polar flagellum. It is distinguished from other *Vibrio* spp. by its ability to ferment lactose. There are two biotypes of *V. vulnificus*. Biotype 1 has an association with human disease (Strom and Paranjpye 2000).

II Health aspects

Primary disease symptoms and sequelae
V. vulnificus is capable of causing necrotising wound infections, gastroenteritis, and primary septicaemia. The symptoms and severity of disease depend on the type of infection. Patients with primary septicaemia usually show symptoms of fever and chills, often with vomiting, diarrhoea and abdominal pain as well as

pain in the extremities. Within the first 24 hours of infection secondary cutaneous lesions appear on the extremities of many patients, including cellulitis, bullae and ecchymosis. Up to 60% of patients experience septicaemic shock with systolic blood pressure below 90 mm Hg. Within seven days about half also experience mental changes. Often the lesions become necrotic and require surgery or amputation. Those who suffer hypotension within 12 hours of admission are at least twice as likely to die compared with those with normal blood pressure (Klontz et al. 1988).

Symptoms shown by patients with V. vulnificus wound infections are similar to those with primary septicaemia, but differ in severity and timing. Most patients report having an acute or pre-existing wound in the week before the onset of illness. The wound becomes inflamed and V. vulnificus can be cultured directly. Wound infections can progress to cellulitis and become necrotic. These patients also often become septicaemic and suffer chills, mental changes, and hypotension. Fatality from wound infections is lower than primary septicaemia, ranging from between 20% and 30% (Strom and Paranjpye 2000).

Most cases of gastroenteritis caused by V. vulnificus are self-limiting and do not require hospitalisation.

Exposure/mechanism of infection

V. vulnificus are opportunistic pathogens causing infection to humans through exposure to seafood and seawater. It is taken up by filter-feeding molluscs and becomes concentrated in the gut and other tissues. Infection occurs through ingestion of contaminated seafood or contact of an open wound with contaminated seawater (Strom and Paranjpye 2000).

Disease incidence

The number of people infected worldwide with V. vulnificus is low compared with other Vibrio spp. (Strom and Paranjpye 2000). The fatality rate ranges from 30% to 75% (Oliver 1989; Anonymous 1996c; Klontz et al. 1998) depending on the mode of infection and the health of the host. Only about 20 deaths per year are reported in the United States from this bacterium (Linkous and Oliver 1999).

Incubation period

Incubation takes up to six days (Patel et al. 2002).

Infectivity

Infectivity is unknown.

Sensitive groups

People with pre-existing liver disease, haematochromatosis, or compromised immune systems are at particularly high risk of fatal septicaemia after ingestion of, or percutaneous exposure to, *Vibrio* spp. (Klontz *et al.* 1988; Levine and Griffin 1993).

III Evidence for association of *Vibrio vulnificus* with recreational waters

Vibrio spp. are natural inhabitants of brackish water and salt water worldwide (Rivera *et al.* 1989; Oliver *et al.* 1995; Montanari *et al.* 1999). *V. vulnificus* is a rare cause of disease, but it is also underreported. The majority of human infections reported in the literature are through consumption of contaminated raw or undercooked seafood. However, infection is also through the contamination of wounds by seawater or marine animals (Hlady and Klontz 1996). One such case of *V. vulnificus* septicaemia, cellulitis and leg ulceration in a patient who had symptoms develop after exposure to brackish water (19 days before admission) or after ingestion of raw oysters (ten days before admission) is described by Patel *et al.* (2002). Recreational water users with open wounds should therefore be aware of the possibility of infection particularly in summer months in temperate areas when the water temperatures are higher.

Between 1997 and 1998, CDC received reports of over 389 cases of culture confirmed *Vibrio* illnesses from the Gulf Coast states, where the majority of cases in the United States have been reported. Among those about whom this information was available, 37% were hospitalised and 7% died. *V. vulnificus* accounted for 89% of the reported deaths. Of the total illnesses reported 16% were classified as wound infections, in which the patient incurred a wound before or during exposure to seawater or seafood drippings, and *Vibrio* spp. was subsequently cultured from the blood, wound or normally sterile site.

There is no national surveillance system in the United States for *V. vulnificus*, but CDC collaborates with the states of Alabama, Florida, Louisiana, Texas and Mississippi to monitor the number of cases of *V. vulnificus* infection in the Gulf Coast region (Evans *et al.* 1999).

Eleven clinical cases of *V. vulnificus* infection occurred in Denmark in the summer of 1994, which was unusually warm (Dalsgaard *et al.* 1996). The route of infection in 10 of the 11 cases was a pre-existing skin lesion. All patients had a history of exposure to seawater or handling of fish prior to infection and none had consumed seafood (Dalsgaard *et al.* 1996). Environmental investigations demonstrated that *V. vulnificus* was prevalent throughout Danish marine environments including coastal water, sediment, wild fish, shellfish and in diseased cultured eels (Høi and Dalsgaard 2000). Four of the patients developed bacteraemia, one of whom died, and nine developed skin lesions.

Anonymous (2003a) Diarrheagenic *Escherichia coli.*
  http://www.cdc.gov/ncidod/dbmd/diseaseinfo/diarrecoli_t.htm.
Anonymous (2003b) Salmonellosis.
  http://www.cdc.gov/ncidod/dbmd/diseaseinfo/salmonellosis_t.htm
Anonymous (2003c) *Shigellosis.*
  http://www.cdc.gov/ncidod/dbmd/diseaseinfo/shigellosis_t.htm.
Anonymous (2004) Legionellosis: Legionnaires' disease and Pontiac fever.
  http://www.cdc.gov/ncidod/dbmd/diseaseinfo/legionellosis_g.htm.
Arean, V.M. (1962) The pathgologic anatomy and pathogenesis of fatal human
  leptospirosis (Weil's disease). *American Journal of Pathology,* **40,** 393–415.
Armengol, S., Domingo, C. and Mesalles, E. (1992) Myocarditis: a rare complication
  during legionella infection. *International Journal of Cardiology*, **37**(3), 418–420.
Armstrong, G.L., Hollingsworth, J. and Morris, J.G. (1996) Emerging food borne
  pathogens: O157:H7 as a model of entry of a new pathogen into the food supply of
  the developed world. *Epidemiologic Reviews*, **18**, 29–51.
Arvanitidou, A., Constantinidis, T.C. and Katsouyannopoulos, V. (1995) A survey on
  Campylobacter and *Yersinia* spp. occurrence in sea and river waters in northern
  Greece. *The Science of the Total Environment,* **171**(1–3, 27), 101–106.
Ashbolt, N. (1996) *Human health risk from microorganisms in the Australian marine
  environment.* Technical Annex 2 of the "State of the Marine Environment Report for
  Australia, 16.
Axelsson-Olsson, D., Waldenstrom, J., Broman, T., Olsen, B. and Holmberg, M. (2005).
  Protozoan *Acanthamoeba polyphaga* as a potential reservoir for *Campylobacter
  jejuni. Applied and Environmental Microbiology*, **71**(2), 987–992.
Barbarino, A. (2002) *Helicobacter pylori*-related iron deficiency anaemia: a review.
  Helicobacter, **7**(2), 71–75.
Barth, W.F. and Segal, K. (1999) Reactive arthritis (Reiters syndrome). *American Family
  Physician,* **60**(2), 499–503.
Barwick, R.S., Levy, D.A., Craun, G.F., Beach, M.J. and Calederon, R.L., (2000)
  Surveillance for waterborne-disease outbreaks – United States, 1997–1998.
  MMWR, **49**(SS04), 1–34.
Bell, B.P., Goldoft, M., Griffin, P.M., Davis, M.A., Gordon, D.C., Tarr, P.I., Bartleson,
  C.A., Lewis, J.H., Barrett, T.J. and Wells, J.G. (1994) A multi-state outbreak of
  Escherichia coli O157:H7-associated bloody diarrhoea and haemolytic uraemic
  syndrome from hamburgers. The Washington experience. *The Journal of the
  American Medical Association,* **272**(17), 1349–1353.
Benkel, D.H., McClure, E.M. Woolard, D., Rullan, J.V., Miller, G.B. Jr., Jenkins, S.R.,
  Hershey, J.H., Benson, R.F., Pruckler, J.M., Brown, E.W., Kolczak, M.S., Hackler,
  R.L., Rouse, B.S and Breiman, R.F. (2000) Outbreak of Legionnaires' disease
  associated with a display whirlpool spa. *International Journal of Epidemiology,*
  29(6), 1092–1098.
Bercovier, H., Kafri, O. and Sela, S. (1986) Mycobacteria possess a surprisingly small
  number of ribosomal RNA genes in relation to the size of their genome.
  Biochemical and Biophysical Research Communications, **136,** 1136–1141.

Bernsen, R.A.J.A.M., Aeiko, E.J., de Jager, P.I., Schmitz, M. and van der Meché, F.G.A. (2002) Long-term impact on work and private life after Guillain–Barré syndrome. *Journal of the Neurological Sciences*, **201**(1–2), 13–17.

Bharti, A.R., Nally, J.E., Ricaldi, J.N., Matthias, M.A., Diaz, M.M., Lovett, M.A., Levett, P.N., Gilman, R.H., Willig, M.R., Gotuzzo, E., Vinetz, J.M., and Peru-United States Leptospirosis Consortium (2003). Leptospirosis: a zoonotic disease of global importance. *The Lancet Infectious Diseases*, **3**(12), 757–771.

Bhopal, R.S. (1993) Geographical variation of Legionnaires' disease: a critique and guide to future research. *International Journal of Epidemiology*, **22**(6), 1127–1136.

Bielaszewska, M., Janda, J., Blahova, K., Minarikova, H., Jikova, E., Karmali, M.A., Laubova, J., Silkulova, J., Preston, M.A., Khakhira, R., Karch, H., Klazarova, H. and Nyc, O. (1997) Human *Escherichia coli* O157:H7 infection associated with the consumption of unpasteurised goat's milk. *Epidemiology and Infection*, **119**, 299–305.

Blaser, M.J., Chyou, P.H. and Nomura, A. (1995) Age at establishment of *Helicobacter pylori* infection and gastric ulcer, and duodenal ulcer risk. *Cancer Research*, **55**, 562–565.

Blostein, J. (1991) Shigellosis from swimming in a park pond in Michigan. *Public Health Reports*, **106**, 317–322.

Bock, B.V., Kirby, B.D., Edelstein, P.H., Snyder, K.M., Hatayama, C.M., Lewis, R.P., George, WL., Owens, ML., Haley, CE., Meyer, RD. and Finegold, SM. (1978) Legionnaires' disease in renal-transplant recipients. *Lancet*, **1**, 410–413.

Bockemuhl, J., Karch, H., Rüssmann, H., Aleksic, S., Wiβ, R. and Emmrich, P. (1990) Shiga-like toxin (Verotoxin)-produzierende *Escherichia coli* O22:H8. *Bundesgesundhbl* (Public Health), **1**, 3–6.

Bode, G., Mauch, F. and Malfertheiner, P. (1993) The coccoid forms of *Helicobacter pylori*. Criteria for their variability. *Epidemiology and Infection*, **111**, 483–490.

Bornstein, N., Marmet, D., Surgot, M., Nowicki, M., Meugnier, H., Fleurette, J., Ageron, E., Grimont, F., Grimont, PAD., Thacker, WL., Benson, RF. and Brenner, D.J. (1989) *Legionella gratiana* sp. nov. isolated from French spa water. *Research in Microbiology*, **140**(8), 541–552.

Brady, M.T. (1989) Nosocomial legionnaires disease in a children's hospital. *Journal of Pediatrics*, **115**(1), 46–50.

Brennan, P.J. and Nikado, H. (1995) The envelope of mycobacteria. *Annual Review of Biochemistry*, **64**, 29–63.

Brennhovd, M., Kapperud, O. and Langeland, G. (1992) Survey of thermotolerant *Campylobacter* spp. and *Yersinia* spp. in three surface water sources in Norway. *International Journal of Food Microbiology*, **15**(3–4), 327–338.

Brewster, D.H., Browne, M.I., Robertson, D., Houghton, G.L., Bimson, J. and Sharp J.C.M. (1994) An outbreak of *Escherichia coli* O157 associated with a children's paddling pool. *Epidemiological Infection*, **112**, 441–447.

Broczyk, A., Thompson, S., Smith, D. and Liorm H. (1987) Waterborne outbreak of *Campylobacter lari* – associated gastroenteritis. *Lancet*, **I**, 164–165.

Brooks, R.W., Parker, B.C. and Falkinham, J.O., III. (1984) Recovery and survival of nontuberculous mycobacteria under various growth and decontamination conditions. *Canadian Journal of Microbiology*, **30**, 1112–1117.

Brutus, J.P., Baeten, Y., Chahidi, N., Kinnen, L., Ledoux, P. and Moermans, J.P. (2001) Atypical mycobacterial infections of the hand: report of eight cases and literature review. *Chirugie de la Main*, **20**, 280–286.

Buzby, J.C. and Roberts T. (1997) Economic and trade impacts of microbial foodborne illness. *World Health Statistical Quarterly*, **50**, 57–66.

Cacciapuoti, L., Ciceroni, A., Pinto, M., Apollini, V., Rondinella, U., Bonomi, E., Benedetti, M., Cinco, S., Dessai, S., Dettori, G., Grillo, R., Falomo, R., Mansueto, S., Miceli, D. and Marcuccio, L. (1994) Survey on the prevalence of Leptospira infections in the Italian population. *European Journal of Epidemiology*, **10**, 173–180.

Calva, E., Torres, J., Vázquez, M., Angeles, V., de la Vega H. and Ruiz-Palacios, G.M. (1989). *Campylobacter jejuni* chromosomal sequences that hybridize to *Vibrio cholerae* and *Escherichia coli*. *Gene*, **75**(2), 243–251.

Cano, R. (1999) Outbreak of Legionnaires' disease associated with a spa resort in Spain. *Eurosurveillance Weekly*, **3**(23), 2.

Carroll, I.M., Khan, A.A. and Ahmed, N. (2004) Revisiting the pestilence of *Helicobacter pylori*: insights into geographical genomics and pathogen evolution, *Infection, Genetics and Evolution*, **4**, 81–90.

Caygill, C.P., Braddick, M., Hill, M.J., Knowles, R.L and Sharp, J.C. (1995) The association between typhoid carriage, typhoid infection and subsequent cancer at a number of sites. *European Journal of Cancer Prevention, The Official Journal of The European Cancer Prevention Organisation*, **4**, 187–193.

CDR (1991) Legionnaires' disease surveillance: England and Wales, 1990. CDR, **1**(6), R65–R66.

CDSC (2000a) Sentinel surveillance of campylobacter in England and Wales. *Communicable Diseases Report Weekly*, **10**(19), 169–172.

CDSC (2000b) *Shigella sonnei* in England and Wales, 1998 and 1999. *Communicable Disease Reports CDR Weekly*, **10**(32), 287.

Chan, E.D., Kong, P.M., Feenelly, K., Dwyer, A.P. and Iseman, M.D. (2001) Vertebral osteomyelitis due to infection with non-tuberculous Mycobacterium species after blunt trauma to the back: 3 examples of the principle of locus minoris resistentiae. *Clinical Infectious Diseases*, **32**, 1506–1510.

Cherry, W.B., Gorman, G.W. Orrison, L.H., Moss, C.W., Steigerwalt, A.G., Wilkinson, H.W., Johnson, S.E., McKinney, R.M and Brenner, D.J. (1982) *Legionella jordanis*: a new species of Legionella isolated from water and sewage. *Journal of Clinical Microbiology*, **15**(2), 290–197.

Ciceroni, L., Stepan, E., Pinto, A., Pizzocaro, P., Dettari, G., Franzin, L., Lupidi, R., Mansueto, S., Manera, A., Iali, A., Marcuccio, L., Grillo, R., Ciarrocchi, S. and Cinco, M. (2000) Epidemiological trend of human leptospirosis in Italy between 1994 and 1996. *European Journal of Epidemiology*, **11**, 707–710.

Clarke, S.C. (2001) Diarrhoeagenic *Escherichia coli* – an emerging problem? *Diagnostic Microbiology and Infectious Disease*, **41**, 93–98.

Cockburne, T.A., Vavra, J.D., Spencer, S.S., Dann, J.R., Peterson, L.J. and Reinhard, K.R. (1954) Human leptospirosis associated with a swimming pool diagnosed after eleven years. *American Journal of Hygiene*, **60**, 1–7.

Colle, I., Van Vlierberghe, H., Troisi, R., De Ridder, K., Benoit, D., de Hemptinne, B. and De Vos, M. (2002) *Campylobacter*-associated Guillain–Barré syndrome after orthotopic liver transplantation for hepatitis C cirrhosis: a case report. *Hepatology Research*, **24**(2), 205–211.

Collier, L., Balows, A. and Sussman, M. (1998) In: *Topley & Wilson's Microbiology and Microbial Infections*. 9th edn., vol. 3 (ed. W.J. Hausler and M. Sussman), pp.421–423. Hodder Arnold.

Collins, C.H., Grange, J.M. and Yates, M.D. (1984) Mycobacteria in water. *Journal of Applied Bacteriology*, **57**(2), 193–211.

Corwin, A., Ryan, A., Bloys, W., Thomas, R., Deniega, B. and Watts, D. (1990) A waterborne outbreak of leptospirosis among United States military personnel in Okinawa, Japan. *International Journal of Epidemiology*, **19**, 743–748.

Covert, T.C., Rodgers, M.R., Reyes, A.L. and Stelma, G.N., Jr. (1999) Occurrence of nontuberculous mycobacteria in environmental samples. *Applied Environmental Microbiology*, **65**, 2492–2496.

Cowden, J.M., Ahmed, S., Donaghy, M. and Riley, A. (2001) Epidemiological investigation of the central Scotland outbreak of *Escherichia coli* O157 infection, November to December 1996. *Epidemiology and Infection*, **126**(3), 335–341.

Cransberg, K., van den Kerkhof, J.H., Banffer, J.R., Stijnen, C., Wernars, K., van de Kar, NC., Nauta, J. and Wolff, E.D. (1996) Four cases of haemolytic uraemic syndrome––source contaminated swimming water? *Clinical Nephrology*, **46**, 45–49.

Van Crevel, R., Speelman, P., Gravekamp, C. and Terpstra, W.J. (1994) Leptospirosis in travellers. *Clinical Infectious Diseases*, **19**, 132–134.

Dalsgaard, A., Frimodt-Møller, N., Bruun, B., Høi, L. and Larsen, J.L. (1996) Clinical manifestations and epidemiology of *Vibrio vulnificus* infections in Denmark. *European Journal of Clinical Microbiology and Infectious Diseases: Official Publication of the European Society of Clinical Microbiology*, **15**(3), 227–231.

Danesh, J., Collins, R. and Peto, R. (1997) Chronic infections and coronary heart disease: is there a link? *Lancet*, **350**(9075), 430–436.

De Brito, T., Beohm, G.M. and Yasuda, P.H. (1979) Vascular damage in acute experimental leptospirosis of the guinea-pig. *Journal of Pathology*, **128**, 177–182.

de Koning, J., van der Hoeven, J.G. and Meinders, A.E. (1995) Respiratory failure in leptospirosis (Weil's disease). *The Netherlands Journal of Medicine*, **47**(5), 224–229.

de Lima, S.C., Sakata, E.E., Santo, C.E., Yasuda, P.H., Stiliano, S.V and Ribeiro, F.A (1990) Outbreak of human leptospirosis by recreational activity in the municipality of Sao Jose dos Campos, Sao Paulo. Seroepidemiological study. *Revista do Instituto de Medicina Tropical de Sao Paulo*, **32**(6), 474–479.

De Luis, D.A., Varela C., De La Calle, H., Canton, R., De Argila, C.M., San Roman, R.L. and Boixeda, D. (1998) *Helicobacter pylori* infection is markedly increased in patients with autoimmune atrophic thyroiditis. *Journal of Clinical Gastroenterology*, **26**(4), 259–263.

De Nileon, G.P. (1998) Water supply implicated in *E. coli* outbreak. Mainstream. *Journal of the American Water Works Association*, **42**, 1.

De Schrijver, K. Dirven, K. Van Bouwel, K., Mortelmans, L., Van Rossom, P., De Beukelaar, T., Vael, C., Fajo, M., Ronveaux, O., Peeters, M.F., Van der Zee, A., Bergmans, A., Ieven, M. and Goossens, H. (2003) An outbreak of Legionnaire's disease among visitors to a fair in Belgium in 1999. *Public Health*, **117**(2), 117–124.

Declercq, J., Verhaegen, J., Verbist, L., Lammens, J., Stuyck, J and Fabry, G. (1994) *Salmonella typhi* osteomyelitis. *Archives of Orthopaedic and Trauma Surgery,* **113,** 232–234.

Delcambre, B., Siame, J.L. and Duquesnoy, B. (1983) The reactive arthritis syndrome. Rheumatological limits. *Revue du Rhumatisme et des Maladies Osteo-Articulaires,* **50**(11), 745–752.

Den Boer, J.W., Jeroen, W. Yzerman, Ed, P.F., Schellekens, J., Lettinga, K.D., Boshuizen, H.C., Van Steenbergen, J.E., Bosman, A., Van den Hof, S., Van Vliet, H.A., Peeters, M.F., Van Ketel, R.J., Ruud, J., Speelman, P., Kool, J.L., Conyn-Van Spaendonck, M.A.E. (2002) A large outbreak of Legionnaires' disease at a flower show, The Netherlands. *Emerging Infectious Diseases,* **8**(1), 37–43.

Den Boer, J.W., Yzerman, E., Van Belkum, A., Vlaspolder, F. and Van Breukelen, F.J. (1998) Legionnaires' disease and saunas. *Lancet,* **351**(9096), 114.

Deschenes, G., Casenave, C., Grimont, F., Desenclos, J.C., Benoit, S., Collin, M., Baron, S., Mariani, P., Grimont, P.A. and Nivet, H. (1996) Cluster of cases of haemolytic uraemic syndrome due to unpasteurised cheese. *Pediatric Nephrology,* **10**(2), 203–205.

Dieu-Osika, S., Tazarourte-Pinturier, S.F., Dessemme, P., Rousseau, P., Sauvion, S., Nathanson, M. and Gaudelus, J. (1996) Encéphalopathie fulminante à *Shigella flexneri. Archives de Pédiatrie,* **3**(10), 993–996.

Domingue, E.L., Tyndall, R.L., Mayberry, W.R. and Pancorbo, O.C. (1988) Effects of three oxidizing biocides on *Legionella pneumophila* serogroup 1. *Applied and Environmental Microbiology,* **54**(3), 741–747.

du Moulin, G.C. and Stottmeister, K.D. (1986) Waterborne mycobacterium: an increasing threat to health. *ASM News,* **52,** 525–529.

Dubois, A. (1995) Spiral bacteria in the human stomach: the gastric helicobacters. *Emerging Infectious Diseases*, **1,** 79–85.

Dufour, A.P. (1984) *Health effects criteria for fresh recreational waters.* Environmental Protection Agency, Cincinnati, USA.

Dunn, B.E., Cohen, H. and Blaser, M.J. (1997) *Helicobacter pylori. Clinical Microbiology Reviews,* **10**(4), 720–741.

Dutka, BJ. and Evans, P. (1986) Isolation of *Legionella pneumophila* from Canadian hot springs. *Canadian Journal of Public Health,* **77**(2), 136–138.

Eyles, R., Niyogi, D., Townsend, C., Benwell, G and Weinstein, P. (2003) Spatial and temporal patterns of Campylobacter contamination underlying public health risk in the Taieri River, New Zealand. *Journal of Environmental Quality,* **32**, 1820–1828.

Edelstein, P.H. and Meyer, R.D. (1984) Legionnaires' Disease: a review. *Chest,* **85**, 114–120.

Edmundson, S.A. and Edmundson, W.C. (1989) Acute diarrhoea disease in India and Indonesia. *Social Science and Medicine,* **29**(8), 991–997.

Elitsur, Y., Btriest, W., Sabet, Z., Neace, C., Jiang, C. and Thomas, E. (2000) Is sudden infant death syndrome associated with *Helicobacter pylori* infection in children? *Helicobacter,* **5**(4), 227–231.

Elliot, E.J., Robins-Browne, R.M., O'Loughlin, E.V., Bennett-Wood, V., Bourke, J., Henning, P., Hogg, G.G., Knight, J. and Powell, H. (2001) Nationwide study of haemolytic uraemic syndrome: clinical, microbiological and epidemiological features. *Archives of Disease in Childhood,* **85**(2), 125–131.

El-Zaatari, F.A.K., Osato, M.S. and Graham, D.Y. (2001) Etiology of Crohn's disease: the role of *Mycobacterium avium paratuberculosis*. *Trends in Molecular Medicine*, 7(6), 247–252.

Embil, J., Warren, P., Yakrus, M., Stark, R., Corne, S. and Forrest, D. (1997) Pulmonary illness associated with exposure to *Mycobacterium avium* complex in hot tub water: hypersensitivity pneumonitis or infection? *Chest*, **111**, 813–816.

Emde, K.M., Chomyc, S.A. and Finch, G.R. (1992) Initial investigation of the occurrence of Mycobacterium species in swimming pools. *Journal of Environmental Health*, **54**, 34–37.

Engstrand, L. (2001) Helicobacter in water and waterborne routes of transmission. *Journal of Applied Microbiology*, **90**, 80S–84S.

Evans, M.C., Griffin, P.M. and Tauxe, R.V. (1999) *Letter to the State and Territorial Epidemiologists concerning the Vibrio surveillance system, summary data, 1997–1998.* Available online. http://www.cdc.gov/ncidod/dbmd/diseaseinfo/cstevib99.pdf. Accessed 14th July 2005.

Evenson, L.J. (1998) Legionnaires' disease. *Primary care update for OB/GYNS*, **5**(6), 286–289.

Fagoonee, S., Pellicano, R., Rizzetto, M. and Pnzetto, A. (2001) The journey from hepatitis to hepatocellular carcinoma. Bridging role of *Helicobacter* species. *Panminerva Medica*, **43**(4), 279–282.

Falkinham, J.O. III, Parker, B.C. and Gruft, H. (1980) Epidemiology of infection by nontuberculous mycobacteria. I. Geographic distribution in the eastern United States. *The American Review of Respiratory Disease*, **121**, 931–937.

Fallon, R.J. and Rowbotham, T.J. (1990) Microbiological investigations into an outbreak of Pontiac fever due to *Legionella micdadei* associated with use of a whirlpool. *Journal of Clinical Pathology*, **43**, 479–483.

Farr, R.W. (1995) Leptospirosis. *Clinical Infectious Diseases*, **21**, 1–8.

Fenlon, DR. (1981) Seagulls (*Larus* spp.) as vectors of salmonella: an investigation into the range of serotype and numbers of salmonellae in gull faeces. *Journal of Hygiene Cambridge*, **86**, 195–202.

Ferguson, C.M., Brian, G., Coote, B.G., Ashbolt, N. and Stevenson, I.M. (1996) Relationships between indicators, pathogens and water quality in an estuarine system. *Water Research*, **30**(9), 2045–2054.

Fewtrell, L., Godfree, A.F., Jones, F., Kay, D., Salmon, R.L. and Wyer, M.D. (1994) *Pathogenic micro-organisms in temperate environmental waters.* Samara Publishing, Cardigan, Dyfed, UK.

Fields, B.S. (1993). Legionella and protozoa: interaction of a pathogen and its natural host, In: *Legionella: current status and emerging perspectives* (ed. J.M. Barbaree, R.F. Breiman, and A.P. Dufour), pp 129–136. American Society for Microbiology, Washington DC, USA.

Fields, B.S., Haupt, T., Davis, J.P., Arduino, M.J., Miller, P.H. and Butler, J.C. (2001) Pontiac fever due to *Legionella micdadei* from a whirlpool spa: possible role of bacterial endotoxin. *Journal of Infectious Diseases*, **184**(10), 1289–1292.

Finegold, S.M. (1988) Legionnaires' disease – still with us. *The New England Journal of Medicine*, **318**(9), 571–573.

Fouad, A., El-Zaatari, K., Osato, M.S. and Graham, D.Y. (2001) Etiology of Crohn's disease: the role of *Mycobacterium avium paratuberculosis*. *Trends in Molecular Medicine,* **7**(6), 247–252.

Frenck, R.W. and Clemens, J. (2003) Helicobacter in the developing world. *Microbes and Infection/Institut Pasteur,* **5**(8), 705–713.

Friedman, M.S., Roels, T., Koehler, J.E., Feldman, L., Bibb, W.F. and Blake, P. (1999) *Escherichia coli* O157:H7 outbreak associated with an improperly chlorinated swimming pool. *Clinical Infectious Diseases: an Official Publication of the Infectious Diseases Society of America,* **29**(2), 298–303.

Gaburri, P.D., Chebli, J.M., de Castro, L.E., Ferreira, J.O., Lopes, M.H., Ribeiro, A.M., Alves, R.A., Froede, E.C., de Oliveira, K.S., Gaburri, A.K., Gaburri, D., Meirelles Gde, S. and de Souza, A.F. (1998) Epidemiology, clinical features and clinical course of Crohn's disease: a study of 60 cases. *Arquivos De Gastrenterologia,* **35**, 240–246.

Galès, P. and Baleux, B. (1992) Influence of the drainage basin input on a pathogenic bacteria (Salmonella) contamination of a Mediterranean lagoon (the Thau lagoon-France) and the survival of this bacteria in brackish water. *Water Science and Technology,* **25**, 105–114.

Gasbarrini, A., Francheshi, F., Cammorata, G., Pola, P. and Gasbarinni, G. (1998) Vascular and immunological disorders associated with *Helicobacter pylori* infection. *Italian Journal of Gastroenterology and Hepatology,* **30**, 115–118.

Gasbarrini, A., Luca, A., Fiore, G., Ojetti, V., Franceschi, F., Di Campli, C., Sanz Torre, E., Candelli, M., Massari, I., Tondi, PP., Serricchio, M., Gasbarrini, G., Pola, P. and Giacovazzo, M. (1997) *Helicobacter pylori* infection: fact and fiction. *Digestive Diseases and Science,* **44**, 229–236.

Geldreich, E.E. (1996) *Microbiological Quality of Water Supply in Distribution Systems.* Lewis Publishers, Boca Raton, USA.

George, K.L. and Falkinham, J.O., III (1986) Selective medium for the isolation and enumeration of *Mycobacterium avium-intracellulare* and *M. scrofulaceum. Canadian Journal of Microbiology,* **32**, 10–14.

George, K.L., Parker, B.C., Gruft, H. and Falkinham, J.O., III. (1980) Epidemiology of infection by nontuberculous mycobacteria. II. Growth and survival in natural waters. *The American Review of Respiratory Disease,* **122**, 89–94.

Ghannem, M., Paule, T., Gabrovescu, M., Menif, W., Meddane, M., Brahimi, K., Marsepoil, T. and Godard, S. (2000) Legionella myopericarditis. *Archives des Maladies du Coeur et des Vaisseaux,* **93**(3), 309–314.

Giesecke, J., Forman, D., Moller, H., Coleman, M. and Eurogast Study Group (1993) An international association between *Helicobacter pylori* and gastric cancer. *Lancet,* **341**(8863), 1359–1362.

Goldberg, D.J., Collier, P.W., Fallon, R.J., McKay, T.M., Markwick, T.A., Wrench, J.G. Emslie, J.A., Forbes, G.I., Macpherson, A.C. and Reid, D. (1989) Lochgilhead fever: outbreak of non-pneumonic legionellosis due to *Legionella micdadei. Lancet,* **1**(8633), 316–318.

Goldwater, P.N. and Bettelheim, K.A. (1995) Hemolytic uremic syndrome due to Shiga-like toxin producing *Escherichia coli* 048:H21 in South Australia. *Emerging Infectious Diseases,* **1**, 132–133.

Goodman, K.J., Correa, P., Aux, H.J.T., Ramirez, H., DeLany, J.P., Pepinosa, O.G., Quinones, M.L. and Parraa, T. (1996) *Helicobacter pylori* infection in the Columbian Andes: a population based study of transmission pathways. *American Journal of Epidemiology,* **144,** 290–299.

Gotz, H.M., Tegnell, A., De Jong, B., Broholm, K.A., Kuusi, M., Kallings, I. and Ekdahl, K. (2001) A whirlpool associated outbreak of Pontiac fever at a hotel in northern Sweden. *Epidemiology and Infection,* **126**(2), 241–247.

Graham, D.Y., Malaty, H.M., Evans, D.G., Evans, D.J., Klein, P.D. and Adam, E. (1991) Epidemiology of *Helicobacter pylori* in an asymptomatic population of the United States. *Gastroenterology,* **100,** 1495.

Gray, J.R. and Rabeneck, L. (1989) Atypical mycobacterial infection of the gastrointestinal tract in AIDS patients. *American Journal of Gastroenterology,* **84,** 1521–1524.

Grennan, S. (1996) Rats alert after death of golfer. *Evening Herald,* August 29, 1.

Grist, N.R., Reid, D. and Najera, R. (1979) Legionnaires' disease and the traveller. *Annals of Internal Medicine,* **90**(4), 563–564.

Groothuis, D.G., Havelaar, A.H. and Veenendaal, H.R. (1985) A note on legionellas in whirlpools. *The Journal of Applied Bacteriology,* **58**(5), 479–481.

Haake, D.A., Dundoo, M., Cader, R., Kubak, B.M., Hartskeerl, R.A., Sejvar, J.J. and Ashford, D.A. (2002). Leptospirosis, water sports and chemoprophylaxis. *Clinical Infectious Diseases,* **34**, 40.

Hartigan, P. (1982) Commentary – leptospirosis in cattle. *Irish Veterinary Journal,* **36,** 180.

Hasselbarth, U. (1992) Prevention of Legionella multiplication in swimming and whirlpools. *Schriftenreihe Des Vereins Fur Wasser-, Boden-Und Lufthygiene,* **91,** 177–181.

Havelaar, A.H., Berwald, L.G., Groothuis, D.G. and Baas, J.G. (1985) Mycobacteria in semi-public swimming pools and whirlpools. *Zentralblatt Fur Bakeriologie Mikrobiologie Und Hygiene,* **180,** 505–514.

Health Canada (2001) Microbial data safety sheets. Available on-line: http://www.hc-sc.gc.ca/pphb-dgspsp/msds-ftss/msds63e.html. Accessed 25th June 2005.

Heath, C.W. Jr., Alexander, A.D. and Galton, M.M. (1965) Leptospirosis in the United States. Analysis of 483 cases in man, 1949, 1961. *The New England Journal of Medicine,* **273**(17), 915–922.

Hegarty, J.P., Dowd, M. and Baker, K.H. (1999) Occurrence of *Helicobacter pylori* in surface waters in the United States. *Journal of Applied Microbiology,* **87,** 697–701.

Helms, C.M., Renner, E.D., Viner, J.P., Hierholzer, W.J.Jr., Winterneyer, L.A. and Johnson, W. (1980) Indirect immunofluorescence antibodies to *Legionella pneumophila*: frequency in a rural community. *Journal of Clinical Microbiology,* **12**(3), 326–328.

Henry, D. and Chamber, R. (2004) Eight hit by bug in swimming pool. http://www.manchesteronline.co.uk/news/s/131/131526_eight_hit_by_bug_in_swimming_pool.html. Accessed 25th November 2004.

Hermon-Taylor, J. (2001) Protagonist. *Mycobacterium avium* subspecies paratuberculous is a cause of Crohn's disease. *Gut,* **49,** 755–756.

Hermon-Taylor, J., Barnes, N., Clarke, C. and Finlayson, C. (1998) Mycobacterium paratuberculosis cervical lymphadenitis, followed five years later by terminal ileitis similar to Crohn's Disease. *British Medical Journal,* **316,** 449–453.

Hermon-Taylor, J., Bull, T.J., Sheridan, J.M., Cheng, J., Stellakis, M.L and Sumar, N., (2000) Causation of Crohn's disease by *Mycobacterium avium* subsp. *paratuberculosis. Canadian Journal of Gastroenterology*, **14,** 521–539.

Hildebrand, S.H., Maguire, H.C., Holliman, R.R. and Kangesu, E. (1996) An outbreak of *Escherichia coli* O157 infection linked to paddling pools. *Communicable Disease Reports Reviews,* **6,** R33–R36.

Hlady, G.W. and Klontz, K. (1996) The epidemiology of vibrio infections in Florida, 1981–1993. *Journal of Infectious Diseases*, **173,** 1176–1183.

Ho, G.Y., Windsor, H.M., Snowball, B. and Marshall, B.J. (2001) *Helicobacter pylori* is not the cause of sudden infant death syndrome (SIDS). *The American Journal of Gastroenterology,* **96**(12), 3288–3294.

Hoffman, S.L., Punjabi, N.H., Kumala, S., Moechtar, M.A., Pulungsih, S.P., Rivai, A.R., Rockhill, R.C., Woodward, T.E and Loedin, A.A. (1984) Reduction of mortality in chloramphenicol-treated severe typhoid fever by high-dose dexamethasone. *New England Journal of Medicine,* **310,** 82–88.

Hoge, C.W. and Breiman, R.F., (1991) Advances in the epidemiology and control of legionella infections. *Epidemiologic Reviews*, **13,** 329–340.

Høi, L. and Dalsgaard, A. (2000) Evaluation of a simplified semi-quantitative protocol for the estimation of *Vibrio vulnificus* in bathing water using cellobiose–colistin agar: a collaborative study with 13 municipal food controlling units in Denmark. *Journal of Microbiological Methods*, **41**(1), 53–57.

Holden, W.S. (1970) *Water Treatment and Examination.* J & A Churchill, London, UK, 248–269.

Holt, J.G., Krieg, N.R., Sneath, P.H.A. and Bergey, D. (1994) *Bergey's Manual of Determinative Bacteriology,* 9th edn., Williams and Wilkins, Baltimore, USA.

Horsburgh, C.R. Jr., Chin, D.P., Yajko, D.M., Hopewell, P.C., Nassos, P.S., Elkin, E.P., Hadley, W.K., Stone, E.N., Simon, E.M. and Gonzalez, P. (1994) Environmental risk factors for acquisition of *Mycobacterium avium* complex in persons with human immunodeficiency virus infection. *Journal of Infectious Diseases,* **170**(2), 362–367.

Horsburgh, C.R. Jr., Gettings, J., Alexander, L.N. and Lennox, J.L. (2001) Disseminated *Mycobacterium avium* complex disease among patients infected with human immunodeficiency virus, 1985–2000. *Clinical Infectious Diseases*, **33**(11), 1938–1943.

Hsu, P.Y., Yang, Y.H., Hsaio, C.H., Lee, P.I. and Chiang, B.L. (2002) *Mycobacterium kasasii* infection presenting as cellulitis in a patient with systemic lupus erythematosus. *Journal of the Formosan Medical Association,* **101**(8), 581–584.

Hulten, K., Enroth, H., Nystrom, T. and Engstrand, L. (1998) Presence of *Helicobacter pylori* species DNA in Swedish water. *Journal of Applied Microbiology*, **85,** 282.

Hulten, K., Han, S.W., Enroth, H., Klein, P.D., Opekun, A.R., Evans, D.G., Engstrand, L., Graham, D.Y. and El-Zaatari, F.A. (1996) *Helicobacter pylori* in the drinking water in Peru. *Gastroenterology*, **110,** 1031–1035.

Hunter, P.R. (1998) *Waterborne Disease Epidemiology and Ecology.* Wiley & Sons Ltd. Chichester, UK.

IASR (2000) Legionellosis, April 1999–July 2000, **21**(9), 186–187.

Iseman, M.D., Corpe, R.F., O'Brien, R.J., Rosenzwieg, D.Y. and Wolinsky, E. (1985) Disease due to *Mycobacterium avium*-intracellulare. *Chest,* **87,** 139S–149S.

Jackson, L.A., Kaufmann, A.F., Adams, W.G., Phelps. M.B., Andreasen, C., Langkop, C.W., Francis, B.J. and Wenger, J.D. (1993) Outbreak of leptospirosis associated with swimming. *Pediatric Infectious Diseases,* **12,** 48–54.

Jennison, A.V. and Verma, N.K. (2004) *Shigella flexneri* infection: pathogenesis and vaccine development. *FEMS Microbiology Reviews,* **28**(1), 43-58

Jeppesen, C., Bagge, L. and Jeppesen, V.F. (2000) *Legionella pneumophila* in pool water. *Ugeskrift for Laeger,* **162**(25), 3592–3594.

Jernigan, D.B., Hofmann, J., Cetron, M.S., Genese, C.A., Nuorti, J.P., Fields, B.S., Benson, R.F., Carter, R.J., Edlestein, P.H., Guerrero, I.C., Paul, S.M., Lipman, H.B. and Breiman, R. (1996) Outbreak of Legionnaires' disease among cruise ship passengers exposed to a contaminated whirlpool spa. *Lancet,* **347**(9000), 494–499.

Johnsen, K., Ostensen, M., Melbye, A.C. and Melby, K. (1983) HLA-B27-negative arthritis related to enteritis in three children and two adults. *Acta Medica Scandinavica,* **214**(2), 165–168.

Johnson, D.C., Enrique, C.E., Pepper, I.L., Davis, T.L., Gerba, C.P., and Rose, J.B. (1997) Survival of Giardia, Cryptosporidium, Poliovirus and Salmonella in marine waters. *Water Science and Technology,* **35**(11–12), 261–268.

Jones, D.L. (1999) Potential health risks associated with the persistence of *E. coli* O157 in agricultural environments. *Soil Use Management,* **15,** 76–83.

Jones, K., Betaieb, M. and Telford, D.R. (1990) Seasonal variation of thermophilic campylobacters in sewage sludge. *Journal of Applied Bacteriology,* **69,** 185–189.

Jones, N.L., Day, A.S. and Sherman, P.M. (1999) Determinants of disease outcome following *Helicobacter pylori* infection in children. *Canadian Journal of Gastroenterology,* **13**(7), 613–617.

Joseph, C.A., Harrison, T.G. and Watson, J.M. (1993) Legionnaires' disease surveillance: England and Wales 1992. *Communicable Disease Report. CDR Review,* **3**(9), R124–R126.

Joseph, C.A., Harrison, T.G. and Watson, J.M. (1994) Legionnaires' disease surveillance: England and Wales, 1993. *Communicable Disease Report. CDR Review,* **4**(10), R109–R112.

Kahana, L.M., Kay, J.M., Yakrus, M.A. and Waserman, S. (1997) *Mycobacterium avium* complex infection in an immunocompetent young adult related to hot tub exposure. *Chest,* **111,** 242–245.

Kaldor, J. and Speed, B.R. (1984) Guillain-Barré syndrome and *Campylobacter jejuni*: a serological study. *British Medical Journal,* **288,** 1867–1870.

Kamimura, M., Katoh, O., Kawata, H., Kudo, K., Yagishita, Y., Niino, H., Saitoh, K., and Saitoh, A. (1998). *Legionella pneumonia* caused by aspiration of hot spring water after sarin exposure. *Journal of the Japanese Respiratory Society,* **36**(3), 278–282.

Karmochkine, M., Cacoub, P., Dorent, R., Laroches, P., Nataf, P., Piette, J.C., Boffa, M.C. and Gandjbakhch, I. (1996) High prevalence of antiphospholipid antibodies in precapillary pulmonary hypertension. *Journal of Rheumatology,* **23,** 286–290.

Katz, A.R., Manea, S.J. and Sasaki, D.M. (1991) Leptospirosis on Kauai: investigation of a common source waterborne outbreak. *American Journal of Public Health,* **81,** 1310–1312.

Keene, W.E., McAnulty, J.M., Hoesly, F.C., Williams, L.P Jr., Hedberg, K., Oxman, G.L., Barrett, T.J., Pfaller, M.A and Fleming, D.W. (1994) A swimming associated outbreak of haemorrhagic colitis caused by *Escherichia coli* O157:H7 and *Shigella sonnei*. *New England Journal of Medicine*, **331**, 579–584.

Khoor, A., Leslie, K.O., Tazelaar, H.D., Hlemers, R.A. and Colby, T.V. (2001) Diffuse pulmonary disease caused by nontuberculous mycobacteria in immunocompetent people (hot tub lung). *American Journal of Clinical Pathology*, **115**, 755–762.

Khosla, S.N. and Lochan, R. (1991) Renal dysfunction in enteric fever. *Journal of Association of Physicians India*, **39**, 382–384.

Kingsley, I., Renee, M.T., Townsend, S.M., Norris, T.L., Ficht, T.A., Adams, L.G and Baumler, A.J. (2000) Impact of horizontal gene transfer on evolution of Salmonella pathogenesis. In: *Virulence Mechanisms of Bacteria Pathogens*, 3rd edition, (ed. K.A. Brogden, J.A. Roth, T.B. Stanton, C.A. Bolin, F.C. Minion, and M.J. Wannemuehler), pp 227–240, ASM Press, Washington, USA.

Kirby, B.D., Synder, K.M., Meyer, R.D. and Finegold, S.M. (1980) Legionnaires' disease: Report of 65 nosocomially acquired cases and review of the literature. *Medicine*, **59**, 188–205.

Kirschener, R.A., Jr., Parker, B.C. and Falkinham, J.O. III. (1992) Epidemiology of infection by nontuberculous mycobacteria. X. *Mycobacterium avium*, *Mycobacterium intracellulare*, and *Mycobacterium scrofulaceum* in acid-brown-water swamps of the south-eastern United States and their association with environmental variables. *The American Review of Respiratory Disease*, **145**, 271–275.

Klein, P.D., Graham, D.Y., Gaillour, A., Opekun, A.R. and Smith, E.O. (1991) Water source as a risk factor for *Helicobacter pylori* infection in Peruvian children. *Lancet*, **337**, 1503–1506.

Klontz, K., Lieb, S., Schreiber, M., Janowski, H., Baldy, L. and Gunn, R. (1988) Syndromes of *Vibrio vulnificus* infections: clinical and epidemiological features in Florida cases, 1981–1987. *Annals of Internal Medicines*, **109**, 318–323.

Konowalchuk, J., Spiers, I. and Satvric, S. (1977) Vero response to a cytotoxin of *Escherichia coli*. *Infection and Immunity*, **18**, 775–779.

Kozin, S.H. and Bishop, A.T. (1994) Atypical Mycobacterium infections of the upper extremity. *Journal of Hand Surgery*, **19**, 480–487.

van Kruiningen, H.J. and Freda, B.J. (2001) A clustering of Crohn's disease in Mankato, Minnesota. *Inflammatory Bowel Disease*, **7**, 27–33.

Kuchta, J.M., States, S.J., McNamara, A.M., Wadowsky, R.M., Yee, R.B. (1983). Susceptibility of *Legionella pneumophila* to chlorine in tap water. *Applied Environmental Microbiology*, **46**, 1134–1139.

Kuipers, E.J., Janssen, M.J.R. and Wink, A. de Boer. (2003). Good bugs and bad bugs: indications and therapies for *Helicobacter pylori* eradication. *Current Opinion in Pharmacology*, **3**(5), 480–485.

Kuntz, T.B. and Kuntz, S.T. (1999) Enterhaemorrhagic *E. coli* infection. *Primary Care Update Ob/Gyns*, **6**(6), 192–195.

Kuroki, S., Saida, T., Nukina, M., Yoshioka, M. and Seino, J. (2001) Three patients with ophthalmoplegia associated with *Campylobacter jejuni*. *Pediatric Neurology*, **25**(1), 71–74.

Kuroki, T., Sata, S., Yamai, S., Yagita, K., Katsube, Y. and Endo, T. (1998) Occurrence of free-living amoebae and Legionella in whirlpool baths. *The Journal of the Japanese Association for Infectious Diseases,* **72**(10), 1056–1063.

Kuth, G., Lamprecht, J. and Haase, G. (1995) Cervical lymphadenitis due to mycobacteria other than tuberculosis – an emerging problem in children? *Journal for Oto-Rhino-Laryngology and its Related Specialities,* **57**, 36–38.

Kuwabara, S., Nakata, M., Sung, J., Mori, M., Kato, N., Hattori, T., Koga, M. and Yuki, N. 2002. Hyperreflexia in axonal Guillain–Barré syndrome subsequent to *Campylobacter jejuni* enteritis. *Journal of the Neurological Sciences,* **199**(1–2), 89–92.

Kvaerner, K.J., Kvestad, E. and Orth, M. (2001) Surgery required to verify atypical mycobacterial infections. *International Journal of Pediatric Otorhinolaryngology,* **61**(2), 121–128.

Laing, R.B.S. (1999) Nosocomial infections in patients with HIV disease. *Journal of Hospital Infection,* **43**(3), 179–185.

Lambert W.C.A., van Breemen, H., Ketelaars, A.M., Hoogenboezem, W. and Medema, G. (1998) Storage reservoirs – a first barrier for pathogenic micro-organisms in The Netherlands. *Water Science and Technology,* **37**(2), 253–260.

Lansbury, L.E. and Ludlam, H. (1997) O157:H7: lessons from the past 15 years. *Journal of Infection,* **34**, 189–193.

Larsson, A., Nilsson, B. and Eriksson, M. (1999) Thrombocytopenia and platelet microvesicle formation caused by *Legionella pneumophila* infection. *Thrombosis Research,* **96**(5), 391–397.

Laurila, A., Bloigu, A., Nayha, S., Hassi, J., Leinonen, M. and Saikku, P. (1999) Association of *Helicobacter pylori* infection with elevated serum lipids. *Atherosclerosis,* **142**, 207–210.

Lawrence, C., Reyrolle, M., Dubrou, S., Forey, F., Decludt, B., Goulvestre, C., Matisota-Bernard, P., Etienne, J. and Nauciel C. (1999) Single clonal origin of a high proportion of *Legionella pneumophila* serogroup 1 isolates from patients and the environment in the rea of Paris, France, over a 10-year-period. *Journal of Clinical Microbiology,* **37**(8), 2652–2655.

Le Saux, N.M., Sekla, L., McLeod, J., Parker, S., Rush, D., Jeffrey, J.R. and Brunham, R.C. (1989) Epidemic of noscomial Legionnaires' disease in renal transplant recipients: a case control and environmental study. *Canadian Medical Association Journal,* **140**, 1047–1053.

Leclerc, H., Schwartzbrod, L. and Dei-Cas, E. (2002) Microbial agents associated with waterborne diseases. *Critical Reviews in Microbiology,* **28**(4), 371–409.

Lee, J.V. and Joseph, C. (2002) Guidelines for investigating single cases of legionnaires' disease. *Communicable Disease and Public Health,* **5**(2), 157–162.

Lee, S.H., Levy, D.A., Craun, G.F., Michael, M.P.H., Beach, J. and Calderon, R.L. (2000a) Surveillance for waterborne-disease outbreaks – United States, 1999–2000. *MMWR,* **51**(SS08), 1–28.

Lee, W.J., Kim, T.W., Shur, K.B., Kook, Y.H., Lee, J.H. and Park, J.K. (2000b) Sporotichoid dermatosis caused by Mycobacterium abscesses from a public bath. *Journal of Dermatology,* **27**(4), 264–268.

Leoni, E., Legnani, P.P., Bucci Sabattini, M.A. and Righi, F. (2001) Prevalence of *Legionella* spp. in swimming pool environment. *Water Research*, **35**(15), 3749–3753.

Levesque, B., Brousseau, P., Bernier, F., Dewailly, E. and Joly, J. (2000) Study of the bacterial content of ring-billed gull droppings in relation to recreational water quality. *Water Research*, **34**(4), 1089–1096.

Levesque, B.B., Brousseau, P., Simard, P., Dewailly, E., Meisels, M., Ramsay, D. and Joly, J. (1993) Impact of the ring-billed gull (*Larus delawarensis*) on the microbiological quality of recreational water. *Applied and Environmental Microbiology*, **59**, 1228–1230.

Levett, P.N. (1999) Leptospirosis: re-emerging or re-discovered disease? *Journal of Medical Microbiology*, **48,** 417–418.

Levine, J.S., Branch, D.W. and Rauch, J. (2002) The antiphospholipid syndrome. *New England Journal of Medicine,* **346,** 752–763.

Levine, W. and Griffin, P. (1993) Vibrio infections on the Gulf Coast: results of first year regional surveillance. *Journal of Infectious Diseases*, **167**, 479–483.

Levy, D., Bens, M.S., Craun, G.F., Calderon, R.L. and Herwaldt, B.L. (1998) Surveillance for waterborne disease outbreaks – United States, 1995–1996. *MMWR,* **47**(SS05), 1–34.

Linkous, D.A. and Oliver, J.D. (1999) Pathogenesis of *Vibrio vulnificus*. *FEMS Microbiology Letters,* **174**(2), 207–214.

Loftus, E.V., Silverstein, M.D., Sandborn, W.J., Tremaine, W.J., Harmsen, S.W. and Zinsmeister, A.R. (1998) Crohn's disease in Olmsted County, Minnesota, 1940–1993: Incidence, Prevalence, and Survival. *Gastroenterology,* **114,** 1161–1168.

Love, W.C., Chaudhuri, A.K., Chin, K.C. and Fallon, R. (1978) Possible case-to-case transmission of Legionnaires' disease. *Lancet,* **2**(8102), 1249.

Loveridge, P. (1981) Legionnaires' disease and arthritis. *Canadian Medical Association Journal*, **124**(4), 366–367.

Lu, Y., Redlinger, T.E., Avitia, R., Galindo, A., and Goodman, K. (2002) Isolation and genotyping of *Helicobacter pylori* from untreated municipal wastewater. *Applied Environmental Microbiology,* **68**, 1436–1439.

Lund, V. (1996) Evaluation of *E. coli* as an indicator for the presence of *Campylobacter jejuni* and *Yersinia enterocolitica* in chlorinated and untreated oligotrophic lake water. *Water Research,* **30**(6), 1528–1534.

Luttichau, H.R., Vinther, C.C., Uldum, S.A., Moller, J., Faber, M. and Jensen, J.S. (1998) An outbreak of Pontiac fever among children following use of a whirlpool. *Clinical Infectious Diseases: an Official Publication of the Infectious Diseases Society of America,* **26**(6), 1374–1378.

Luttichau, H.R., Vinther, C.C., Uldum. S.A. Moller, J.S., Faber, M. and Jensen, J.S. (1999) An outbreak of Pontiac fever among children and adults following a whirlpool bath. *Ugeskrift for Laeger,* **161**(23), 3458–3462.

Mahon, B.E., Griffin, P.M., Mead, P.S. and Tauxe, R.V. (1997) Haemolytic uraemic syndrome surveillance to monitor trends in infection with *Escherichia coli* O157:H7 and other Shiga toxin-producing *E. coli*. *Emerging Infectious Diseases,* **3**(3), 409–412.

Makintubee, S., Mallonee, J. and Istre GR. (1987) Shigellosis outbreak associated with swimming. *American Journal of Public Health,* **77,** 166–168.

Mamane, M., Kasparian, P., Babo, P. and Accard, J.L. (1983) Legionnaires' disease with late pulmonary sequelae. Apropos of a case. *Le Poumon et le Coeur,* **39**(6), 305–308.

Mandell, G.L., Douglas, R.G and Bennett, J.E. (1990) *Principles and Practice of Infectious Diseases.* Churchill Livingstone, New York, United States.

Mangione, E.J., Huitt, G., Lenaway, D., Beebe, J., Bailey, A., Figoski, M., Rau, M.P., Albrecht, K.D. and Yakrus, M.A. (2001) Nontuberculous mycobacterial disease following hot tub exposure. *Emerging Infectious Diseases,* **7**(6), 1039–1042.

Mangione, E., Remis, R.S., Tait, K.A., McGee, H.B., Gorman, G.W., Wentworth, B.B., Baron, P.A., Hightower, A.W., Barbaree, J.M. and Broome, C.V. (1985) An outbreak of Pontiac fever related to whirlpool use, Michigan 1982. *Journal of the American Waterworks Association,* **253**(4), 535–539.

Marras, T.K. and Daley, C.L. (2002) Epidemiology of human pulmonary infection with nontuberculous mycobacteria. *Clinics in Chest Medicine,* **23,** 553–567.

Marston, B.J., Lipman, H.B. and Breiman, R.F. (1994) Surveillance for Legionnaires' disease. Risk factors for morbidity and mortality. *Archives of Internal Medicine,* **154**(21), 2417–2422.

Martin, D., MacDonald, K., White, K., Soler, J. and Osterholm, M. (1990) The epidemiology and clinical aspects of the hemolytic uremic syndrome in Minnesota. *New England Journal of Medicine,* **323,** 1161–1167.

Martinelli, F., Carasi, S., Scarcella, C. and Speziani, F. (2001) Detection of *Legionella pneumophila* at thermal spas. *The New Microbiologica: Official Journal of the Italian Society for Medical, Odontoiatric, and Clinical Microbiology (SIMMOC),* **24**(3), 259–264.

Mashiba, K., Hamamoto, T. and Torikai, K. (1993) A case of Legionnaires' disease due to aspiration of hot spring water and isolation of *Legionella pneumophila* from hot spring water. *The Journal of the Japanese Association for Infectious Diseases,* **67**(2), 163–166.

Mazari-Hiriart, M., López-Vidal, Y., Castillo-Rojas, G., Ponce de León, S. and Cravioto, A. (2001) *Helicobacter pylori* and other enteric bacteria in freshwater environments in Mexico City. *Archives of Medical Research,* **32**(5), 458–467.

McDonald, S.D. and Gruslin, A. (2001) A review of *Campylobacter* infection during pregnancy: a focus on *C. jejuni. Primary Care Update for OB/GYNS,* **8**(6), 253–257.

McEvoy, M., Batchelow, N., Hamilton, G., MacDonald, A., Faiers, M., Sills, A., Lee, J. and Harrison, T. (2000) A cluster of cases of Legionnaires' disease associated with exposure to a spa pool on display. *Communicable Disease and Public Health/PHLS,* **3**(1), 43–45.

Medema, G.J., van Asperen, I.A., Klokman-Houweling, J.M., Nooitgedagt, A., van de Laar, W. and Havelaar, A.H. (1995) The relationship between health effects in triathletes and microbiological quality of freshwater. *Water Science and Technology,* **31**(5–6), 19–26.

Megraud, F., Brassens rabbe, M.P, Denis, F., Belbouri, A. and Hoa, D.Q. (1989) Seroepidemiology of Campylobacter pylori infection in various populations. *Journal of Clinical Microbiology,* **27,** 1870-1873.

Merat, S., Malekzadeh, R., Varshosaz, J., Sotoudehmanesh, R. and Agah, S. (2002) Crohn's disease in Iran: A report of 140 cases. *Gut,* **51,** A128.

Mery, A. and Horan, R.F. (2002) Hot tub-related *Mycobacterium avium* intracellulare pneumonitis. *Allergy and Asthma Proceedings: The Official Journal of Regional and State Allergy Societies,* **23,** 271–273.

Mijs, W., de Haas, P., Rossau, R., Van Der Laan, T., Rigouts, L., Portaels, F. and van Soolingen, D. (2002) Molecular evidence to support a proposal to reserve the designation *Mycobacterium avium* subsp. *avium* for bird-type isolates and *M. avium* subsp. *hominissuis'* for the human/porcine type of *M. avium. International Journal of Systematic and Evolutionary Microbiology,* **52,** 1505–1518.

Miller, L.A. and Beebe, J.L. (1993) Use of polymerase chain reaction in an epidemiologic investigation of Pontiac fever. *The Journal of Infectious Diseases,* **168**(3), 769–772.

Minnesota Department of Health (1974) An outbreak of shigellosis associated with lake swimming; southwestern Minnesota, June 1994. *Disease Control Newsletter,* **22,** 45–46.

Mishu, B., Patton, C.M. and Tauxe, R.V. (1992) Clinical epidemiologic features of non-jejuni, non-coli *Campylobacter* species. In: *Campylobacter jejuni: current status and future trends* (ed. I. Namchamkin, M.J. Blaser and L.S. Tompkins), pp.31–41 American Society for Microbiology Press, Washington, USA.

Miwa, H., Sakaki, N., Sugiyama, T. and Helicobacter Forum of Japan (2002) Incidence of recurrent peptic ulcers in patients with cured *H. pylori* infection – a large-scale multicenter study from Japan. *The American Journal of Gastroenterology,* **97**(9, Supplement 1), S42.

Miyamoto, M., Yamaguchi, Y. and Sasatsu, M. (2000) Disinfectant effects of hot water, ultraviolet light, silver ions and chlorine on strains of *Legionella* and nontuberculous mycobacteria. *Microbios,* **101,** 7–13.

Molmeret, M., Jarraud, S., Mori, J.P., Pernin, P., Forey, F., Reyrolle, M., Vandenesch, F., Etienne, J. and Farge, P. (2001) Different growth rates in ameoba of genotypically related environmental and clinical *Legionella pneumophila* strains isolated from a thermal spa. *Epidemiology and Infection,* **126**(2), 231–239.

Montanari, M.P., Pruzzo, C., Pane, L. and Colwell, R.R. (1999) Vibrios associated with plankton in a coastal zone of the Adriatic Sea (Italy). *FEMS Microbiology Ecology,* **29**(3), 241–247.

Moreno, Y., Ferrús, M.A., Alonso, J.L., Jiménez, A. and Hernández, J. (2003) Use of fluorescent in situ hybridization to evidence the presence of *Helicobacter pylori* in water. *Water Research,* **37**(9), 2251–2256.

Motes, M.L., De Paola, A., Cook, D.W., Veazey, J.E., Hunsucker, J.C., Garthright, W.E., Blodgett, R.J. and Chirtel, S.J. (1998) Influence of water temperature and salinity on *Vibrio vulnificus* in Northern Gulf and Atlantic Coast oysters *(Crassostrea virginica). Applied Environmental Microbiology,* **64,** 1459.

Mou, S.M. (1998) The relationship between Helicobacter infection and peptic ulcer disease. *Infectious Disease Update,* **5**(5), 229–232.

Murakami, K., Jujjoka, T., Nishizono, A., Nagai, J., Tokeida, M., Kodama, R., Kubota, T. and Nasu, M. (1996) Atopic dermatitis successfully treated by eradication of *Helicobacter pylori. Journal of Gastroenterology,* **31**(9), 77–82.

Nachamkin, I. (2002) Chronic effects of *Campylobacter* infection. *Microbes and Infection,* **4**(4), 399–403.

Nakadate, T., Yamauchi, K. and Inoue, H. (1999) An outbreak of Legionnaires' disease associated with a Japanese spa. *Journal of the Japanese Respiratory Society,* **37**(8), 601–607.

Nataro, J.P. and Kaper, J.B. (1998) Diarrhoeagenic *Escherichia coli. Clinical Microbiology Reviews,* **11**(1), 142–201.

Newman, C.P.S. (1993) Surveillance and control of *Shigella sonnei* infection. *CDR Review,* **3**(5), R63–R70.

Newman, R.D., Wuhib, T., Lima, A.A.M., Guerrant, R.L. and Sears, C.L. (1993) Environmental sources of *Cryptosporidium* in an urban slum in northeastern Brazil. *American Journal of Tropical Medicine and Hygiene,* **49,** 270–275.

Newsome, A.L., Baker, R.L., Miller, R.D. and Arnold, R.R. (1985) Interactions between *Naegleria fowleri* and *Legionella pneumophila. Infection and Immunity,* **50**(2), 449–452.

Nguyen, M.H., Stout, J.E. and Yu, V.L. (1991) Legionellosis. *Infectious Disease Clinics of North America,* **5**(3), 561–584.

Nguyen, T.N., Barkin, A.N. and Fallone, C.A. (1999) Host determinants of *Helicobacter pylori* infection and its clinical outcome. *Helicobacter,* **4**(3), 185–197.

Nicodema, A.C., Medeiros, N., del Negro, G. and Amato Neto, V. (1989) Haematologic changes in leptospirosis. *Revista Do Instuto De Medicina Tropical De Sao Paulo,* **31**(2), 71–79.

Nizeyi, J.B., Innocent, R.B., Erume, J., Kalema, G.R.N.N., Cranfield, R.M. and Graczyk, T.K. (2001) Campylobacteriosis, salmonellosis, and shigellosis infections in free-ranging human-habituated gorillas of Uganda. *Journal of Wildlife Diseases,* **37,** 239–244.

O'Brien, R.J., Geiter, L. and Snider, D.E. (1987) The epidemiology of non-tuberculous mycobacterial diseases in the United States. *The American Review of Respiratory Disease,* **135,** 1007–1014.

Obiri-Danso, K. and Jones, K. (1999) The effect of a new sewage treatment plant on faecal indicator numbers, *campylobacters* and bathing water compliance in Morecambe Bay. *Journal of Applied Microbiology,* **86,** 603–614.

Obiri-Danso, K. and Jones, K. (2000) Intertidal sediments as reservoirs for hippurate negative campylobacters, salmonellae and faecal indicators in three EU recognised bathing waters in north west England. *Water Research,* **34**(2), 519–527.

Oldenburg, B., Diepersloot, R.J.A. and Hoekstra, J.B.L. (1996) High seroprevalence of *Helicobacter pylori* in diabetes mellitus patients. *Digestive Diseases and Science,* **41,** 458–461.

Oliver, J.D. (1989) *Vibrio vulnificus.* In: *Foodborne Bacterial Pathogens,* (ed. M.P. Doyle), pp. 569–599. Marcel Dekker, New York, USA.

Oliver, J.D. (1995) The viable but non-culturable state in the human pathogen *Vibrio vulnificus. FEMS Microbiology Letters,* **133**(3), 203–208.

Ortiz-Roque, C.M. and Hazen, T.C. (1987) Abundance and distribution of Legionellaceae in Puerto Rican waters. *Applied and Environmental Microbiology,* **53**(9), 2231–2236.

Pai, C.G. and Khandige, G.K. (2000) Is Crohn's disease rare in India? *Indian Journal of Gastroenterology,* **19,** 17–20.

Palmer, C.J., Tsai, Y.L., Paszko-Kolva, C., Mayer, C. and Sangermano, L.R. (1993) Detection of *Legionella* species in sewage and ocean water by polymerase chain reaction, direct fluorescent-antibody, and plate culture methods. *Applied and Environmental Microbiology*, **59**(11), 3618–3624.

Pang, T., Levine, M.M., Ivanoff, B., Wain J. and Finlay, B.B. (1998) Typhoid fever – important issues still remain. *Trends in Microbiology*, **6**(4), 131–133.

Park, S. (2002) The physiology of *Campylobacter* species and its relevance to their role as foodborne pathogens. *International Journal of Food Microbiology*, **74**(3), 177–188.

Parker, M.T. (1990) Enteric infections: typhoid and paratyphoid. In: Topley & Wilson's *Principles of Bacteriology, Virology and Immunity*, vol. 3, 8th edn. (ed. M.T. Parker, and L.H. Collier), pp 424–46, Edward Arnold, London, UK.

Parsonnet, J. (1995) The incidence of *Helicobacter pylori* infection. *Alimentary Pharmacology and Therapeutics*, **9**(2), 45–51.

Parsonnet, J., Harris, R.A., Hack, H.M. and Owens, D.K. (1996) Modelling cost-effectiveness of *Helicobacter pylori* screening to prevent gastric cancer: A mandate for clinical trials. *Lancet*, **348**(9021), 758–759.

Patel, V.J., Gardner, M.D. and Burton, C.S. (2002) *Vibrio vulnificus* septicaemia and leg ulcer. *Journal of the American Academy of Dermatology*, **46**(5 part 2), S144–S145.

Patterson, W.J., Seal, D.V., Curran, E., Sinclaie, T.M. and McLuckie, J.C. (1994) Fatal nosocomial Legionnaires' disease: relevance of contamination of hospital water supply by temperature-dependent buoyancy-driven flow from spur pipes. *Epidemiology and Infection*, **112**(3), 513–525.

Pattison, C.P., Marshall, B.J., Young, T.W., Vergara, G.C., Smith, G.P. and Case, M.E. (1997) Prevalence of *Helicobacter pylori* (HP) in SIDS/non SIDS autopsies (abstract). *Journal of Pediatric Gastroenterology and Nutrition*, **25**, 467.

Peliowski, A. and Finer, N.N. (1986) Intractable seizures in Legionnaires' disease. *The Journal of Pediatrics*, **109**(4), 657–658.

PHLS (1959) Sewage contamination of coastal bathing water in England and Wales. A bacteriological and epidemiological study. By the Committee of the Public Health Laboratory Service. *Journal of Hygiene*, **57,** 435–472.

Pianetti, A., Baffone, W., Bruscolini, F., Barbieri, E., Biffi, M.R., Salvaggio, L. and Albano, A. (1998) Presence of several pathogenic bacteria in the Metauro and Foglia Rivers (Pesaro-Urbino, Italy). *Water Research*, **32**(5), 1515–1521.

Pickles, J., Feakins, R.M., Hansen, J., Sheaff, M. and Barnes, N. (2001) A case of *Mycobacterium avium-intracellulare* pulmonary disease and Crohn's disease. *Grand Rounds*, **2**, 24–28.

Plank, R. and Dean, D. (2000) Overview of the epidemiology, microbiology, and pathogenesis of *Leptospira* spp. in humans. *Microbes and Infection*, **2,** 1265–1276.

Polo, F., Figueras, M.J., Inza, I., Sala, J., Fleisher, J.M. and Guarro, J. (1998) Relationship between presence of *Salmonella* and indicators of faecal pollution in aquatic habitats. *FEMS Microbiology Letters*, **160**(2), 253–256.

Popoff, M.Y., Bockemuhl, J. and Brenner, F.W. (2000) Supplement 1998 (no.42) to the Kuffmann-White scheme. *Research in Microbiology*, **151,** 63–65.

Pozniak, A. and Bull, T. (1999) Recently recognised mycobacteria of clinical significance. *Journal of Infection*, **38**(3), 157–161.

Proctor, M.E. and Davis, J.P. (2000) *Escherichia coli* 0157:H7 infections in Wisconsin, 1992–1999. *WMJ: Official Publication of the State Medical Society of Wisconsin*, **99**(5), 32–37.

Rastogi, N., Frehel, C., Ryter, A., Ohayon, H., Lesourd, M. and David, H.L. (1981) Multiple drug resistance in *Mycobacterium avium*: is the wall archeitecture responsible for the exclusion of antimicrobial agents? *Antimicrobial Agents and Chemotherapy,* **20,** 666–667.

Realdi, G., Dore, M.P.and Fastame, L. (1999) Extradigestive manifestations of *Helicobacter pylori* infection: fact and fiction. *Digestive Diseases and Science,* **44,** 229–236.

Rickman, O.B., Ryu, J.H., Fidler, M.E. and Kalra, S. (2002). Hypersensitivity pneumonitis associated with *Mycobacterioum avium* complex and hot tub use. *Mayo Clinic Proceedings,* **11,** 1233–1237.

Rivera, S., Lugo, T. and Hazen, T.C. (1989) Autecology of *Vibrio vulnificus* and *Vibrio parahaemolyticus* in tropical waters. *Water Research,* **23**(7), 923–931.

Robinson, D.A. (1981) Infective dose of *Campylobacter jejuni* in milk. *British Medical Journal,* **282,** 1584.

Roig, J., Carreres, A. and Domingo, C. (1993) Treatment of Legionnaires' disease. Current recommendations. *Drugs,* **46**(1), 63–79.

Rollins, D. and Colwell, R. (1986) Viable but non-culturable stage of *Campylobacter jejuni* and its role in survival in the natural aquatic environment. *Applied and Environmental Microbiology,* **52**(3), 531–538.

Rose, C.S., Martyny, J.W., Newman, L.S., Milton, D.K., King, T.E. Jr., Beebe, J.L., McCammon, J.B., Hoffman, R.E. and Kreiss, K. (1998) 'Lifeguard Lung': Endemic granulomatous pneumonitis in an indoor swimming pool. *American Journal of Public Health,* **88,** 1795–1800.

Rosenberg, M.L., Hazlet, K.K., Schaefer, J., Wells, J.G. and Pruneda, R.C. (1976) Shigellosis from swimming. *Journal of the American Medical Association,* **236,** 1849–1852.

Rothenbacher, D. and Brenner, H. (2003) Burden of *Helicobacter pylori* and *H. pylori*-related diseases in developed countries: recent developments and future implications. *Microbes and Infection,* **5**(8), 339–345.

Rowe, P.C., Orrbine, E., Lior, H., Wells, G.A., Yetisir, E., Clulow, M. and McLaine, P.N. (1998) Risk of haemolytic uraemic syndrome after sporadic O157:H7 infection: Results of a Canadian collaborative study. *The Journal of Pediatrics,* **132,** 777–782.

Rowe, P.C., Orrbine, E., Wells, G.A. and McLaine, P.N. (1991) Epidemiology of haemolytic-uraemic syndrome in Canadian children from 1986 to 1988. *The Journal of Pediatrics,* **119**(2), 218–224.

Rowland, R. and Drumm, B. (2001) *Helicobacter pylori* and sudden-infant-death syndrome. *Lancet,* **357**(9253), 327.

Rugman, F.P., Pinn, G., Palmer, M.F., Waite, M. and Hay, C.R. (1991) Anticardiolipin antibodies in leptospirosis. *Journal of Clinical Pathology,* **44,** 517–519.

Rusin, P.A., Rose, J.B., Haas, C.N. and Gerba, C.P. (1997) Risk assessment of opportunistic bacterial pathogens in drinking water. *Reviews of Environmental Contamination and Toxicology,* **152,** 57–83.

Sanford, J.P. (1979) Current concepts of Legionnaires' disease – a clarification. *The New England Journal of Medicine,* **301**(5), 277.

Seidel, K. (1987) Presence of *Legionella pneumophila* in drinking water and water from warm spring pools. *Schriftenreihe Des Vereins Fur Wasser-, Boden und Lufthygiene*, **72**, 67–75.

Shaffler-Dullnig, K., Reinthaler, F.F. and Marth, E. (1992) Detection of legionellae in thermal water. *International Journal of Hygiene and Environmental Medicine*, **192**(5), 473–478.

Shahamat, M., Mai, U., Paszko-Kolva, C.P., Kessel, M. and Colwell, R.R. (1993) Use of autoradiography to assess viability of *Helicobacter pylori* in water. *Applied Environmental Microbiology*, **59**, 1231–1235.

Shelton, B.G., Flanders, W.D. and Morris, G.K. (1999) *Mycobacterium sp.* as a possible cause of hypersensitivity pneumonitis in machine workers. *Emerging Infectious Diseases*, **5**(2), 270–273.

Shiraishi, Y., Nakaima, Y., Takasuna, K., Hanaoka, T., Katsuragi, N. and Konno, H. (2002) Surgery for *Mycobacterium avium* complex lung disease in the clarithromycin era. *European Journal of Cardio-Thoracic Surgery: Official Journal of the European Association for Cardio-Thoracic Surgery*, **21**, 314–318.

Shpilberg, O., Shaked, Y., Maier, M.K., Samra, D. and Samra, Y. (1990) Long term follow-up after leptospirosis. *Southern Medical Journal*, **83**, 405–407.

Siegler, R., Pavia, A., Christofferson, R. and Milligan M. (1994) A 20-year population-based study of postdiarrhoeal haemolytic uraemic syndrome in Utah. *Pediatrics*, **96**, 35–40.

Skirrow, M.B. (1990) *Campylobacter. Lancet*, **336**(8720), 921–923.

Skirrow, M.B. (1991) Epidemiology of *Campylobacter* enteritis. *International Journal of Food Microbiology*, **12**(1), 9–16.

Skirrow, M.B. and Blaser, M.J. (2000) In: *Campylobacter* (ed. I. Nachamkin and M.J. Blaser), pp. 69–88, American Society for Microbiology Press, Washington, USA.

Slutsker, L., Ries, A.A., Greene, K.D., Wells, J.G., Hutwagner, L. and Griffin P.M. (1997) *Escherichia coli* O157:H7 diarrhoea in the United States: clinical and epidemiologic features. *Annals of Internal Medicine*, **126**(7), 505–513.

Smeal, W.E., Scehfeld, L.A., and Hauger, W. (1985) *Legionella* causing rhabdomyolysis and renal failure. *Postgraduate Medicine*, **78**(2), 42–44.

Solnick J.V., Hansen, L.M., Canfield, D.R. and Parsonnet, J. (2001) Determination of the infectious dose of *Helicobacter pylori* during primary and secondary infection with Rhesus Monkeys (*Macca mulatta*). *Infections and Immunity*, **69**(11), 6887–6892.

Somers, C.J., Al-Kindi, S., Montague, S., O'Connor, R., Murphy, P.G., Jeffers, M. and Enright, H. (2003) Erythroid hypolasia associated with leptospirosis. *Journal of Infection*, **47**(1), 85–86.

Sommese, L., Scarfogliero, P., Vitiello, M., Catalanotti, P. and Galdiero, E. (1996) Presence of *Legionella* spp. in thermal springs of the Campania region of south Italy. *The New Microbiologica: Official Journal of the Italian Society for Medical, Odontoiatric, and Clinical Microbiology (SIMMOC)*, **19**(4), 315–320.

Sorvillo, F.J., Lieb, L.E. and Waterman, S.H. (1991) Incidence of campylobacteriosis among patients with AIDS in Los Angeles County. *Journal of Acquired Immune Deficiency Syndrome*, **4**(6), 598–602.

Sorvillo, F.J., Waterman, S.H., Vogt, J.K. and England, B. (1988) Shigellosis associated with recreational water contact in Los Angeles County. *American Journal of Tropical Medicine and Hygiene*, **38**, 613–617.

Spitalny, K.C., Vogt, R.L., Orciari, L.A., Witherell, L.E., Etkind, P. and Novick, L.F. (1984) Pontiac fever associated with a whirlpool. *American Journal of Epidemiology,* **120**(6), 809–817.

Strachan, D.P. (1998) Non-gastrointestinal consequences of *Helicobacter pylori* infection. *British Medical Bulletin,* **54**(1), 87–93.

Surman, S., Lee, J.V., Pond, K.R., Chartier, Y. and Bartram, J. (2005) *Legionella and the prevention of legionellosis.* WHO, Geneva. In Press.

van Basten, J.P. and Stockenbrugger, R. (1994) Typhoid perforation. A review of the literature since 1960. *Tropical and Geographical Medicine,* **46**, 336–339.

van Steenbergen, J.E., Slijkerman, F.A.N. and Speelman, P. (1999) The first 48 hours of investigation and intervention of an outbreak of legionellosis in the Netherlands. *Eurosurveillance Monthly,* **4**(11), 111–115.

von Reyn, C.F., Waddell, R.D., Eaton, T., Arbeit, R.D., Maslow, J.N., Barber, T.W., Brindle, R.J., Gilks, C.F., Lumio, J., Lahdevirta, J., Ranki, A., Dawson, D. and Falkinham, J.O. III. (1993) Isolation of *Mycobacterium avium* complex from water in the United States, Finland, Zaire, and Kenya. *Journal of Clinical Microbiology,* **31**, 3227–3230.

Strom, M.S. and Paranjpye, R.N. (2000) Epidemiology and pathogenesis of *Vibrio vulnificus. Microbes and Infection,* **2**(2), 177–188.

Sugita, T., Ishii, N., Katsuno, M., Yamada, R. and Nakajima, H. (2000) Familial cluster of cutaneous *Mycobacterium avium* infection resulting from use of a circulating, constantly heated bath water system. *British Journal of Dermatology,* **142**(4), 789–793.

Swerdlow, D.L., Woodruff, B.A., Brady, R.C., Griffin, P.M., Tippen, S., Donnel, H.D., Geldreich, E., Payne, B.J., Meyer, A. and Wells, J.G. (1992) A waterborne outbreak in Missouri of *Escherichia coli* O157:H7 associated with bloody diarrhoea and death. *Annals of Internal Medicine,* **117**(7), 812–819.

Talibart, R., Denis, M., Castillo, A., Cappelier, J.M. and Ermel, G. (2000) Survival and recovery of viable but noncultivable forms of Campylobacter in aqueous microcosm. *International Journal of Food Microbiology,* **55**(1–3), 263–267.

Tarr, P.I. and Hickman, R.O. (1987) Hemolytic uremic syndrome epidemiology: A population-based study in King Country, Washington, DC and Baltimore, Maryland. *American Journal of Public Health,* **78**, 64–65.

Tattevin, P., Dupeux, S. and Hoff, J. (2003) Leptospirosis and the antiphospholipid syndrome. *The American Journal of Medicine,* **114**(2), 164.

Taviot, B., Gueyffier, F., Pacheco, Y., Boniface, E., Coppere, B. and Perrin-Fayolle, M. (1987) Purulent pleurisy due to *Legionella bozemanii. Revue des Maladies Respiratoires,* **4**(1), 47–48.

Taylor, R.H., Falkinham, J.O., III, Norton, C.D. and LeChevallier, M.W. (2000) Chlorine, chloramine, chlorine dioxide, and ozone susceptibility of *Mycobacterium avium. Applied Environmental Microbiology,* **66**, 1702–1705.

Thi Minh Chau, L.Y. and Muller, H.E. (1983) Incidence of Legionnaires' disease. *Deutsche Medizinishche Wochenschrift,* **108**(40), 1508–1511.

Thiermann, A.B. (1977) Incidence of leptospirosis in the Detroit rat population. *American Journal of Tropical Medical and Hygiene,* **26**, 770–774.

Thomas, J.E., Dale, A., Harding, M., Coward, W.A., Cole, T.J. and Weaver, L.T. (1999) *Helicobacter pylori* colonization in early life. *Pediatric Research,* **45**, 218–223.

Tison, D.L., Pope, D.H., Cherry, W.B. and Fliermans, C.B. (1980) Growth of *Legionella pneumophila* in association with blue-green algae (cyanobacteria). *Applied and Environmental Microbiology*, **39**(2), 456–459.

Tokuda, H., Yahagi, N., Kasai, S., Kitamura, S. and Otsuka, Y. (1997) A case of fatal pneumonia caused by *Legionella pneumophila* serogroup 6 developed after drowning in a public bath. *The Journal of the Japanese Association for Infectious Diseases*, **71**(2), 169–179.

Tolentino, A., Ahkee, S. and Ramirez, J. (1996) Hot tub legionellosis. *The Journal of the Kentucky Medical Association*, **94**(9), 393–394.

Tominaga, M., Aoki, Y., Haraguchi, S., Fukuoka, M., Hayashi, S., Tamesada, M., Yabuuchi, E. and Nagasawa, K. (2001) Legionnaires' disease associated with habitual drinking of hot spring water. *Internal Medicine*, **40**(10), 1064–1067.

Tomov, A., Tsvetkova, E., Tsanev, N., Kassovsky, V. and Gotev, N. (1981) Isolation of *Legionella pneumophila* in Bulgaria. *International Journal of Microbiology and Hygiene. A, Medical Microbiology*, **250**(4), 521–528.

Torre, D., Giola, M., Martegani, R., Zeroli, C., Fiori, G.P., Ferrario, G. and Bonetta, G. (1994) Aseptic meningitis caused by *Leptospira australis*. *European Journal of Clinical Microbiology and Infectious Diseases*, **13**, 496–497.

Trevejo, R.T., Rigau-Perez, J.G., Ashford, D.A., McClure, E.M., Jarquain-Gonzaalez, C., Amador, J.J., De Los Reyes, J.O., Gonzalez, A., Zaki, S.R., Shieh, W.J., McLean, R.G., Nasci, R.S., Weyant, R.S., Bolin, C.A., Bragg, S.L., Perkins, B.A. and Spiegel, R.A. (1995) Epidemic leptospirosis associated with pulmonary haemorrhage – Nicaragua. *Journal of Infectious Diseases*, **178**, 1457–1463.

Trupiano, J.K. and Prayson, R.A. (2001) *Mycobacterium avium intracellulare* otitis media. *Annals of Diagnostic Pathology*, **5**(6), 350–353.

van Bohemen, Ch. G., Nabbe, A. J. J. M., Dinant, H. J., Grumet, F. C., Landheer, J. E. and Zanen, H.C. (1986) Lack of serologically defined arthritogenic *shigella flexneri* cell envelope antigens in post-dysenteric arthritis. *Immunology Letters*, **13**(4), 197–201.

Velázquez, M. and Feirtag, J.M. (1999) *Helicobacter pylori*: characteristics, pathogenicity, detection methods and mode of transmission implicating foods and water. *International Journal of Food Microbiology*, **53**(2–3), 95–104.

Verissimo, A., Marrao, G., da Silva, F.G. and da Costa, M.S. (1991) Distribution of *Legionella* spp. in hydrothermal areas in continental Portugal and the island of Sao Miguel, Azores. *Applied and Environmental Microbiology*, **57**(10), 2921–2927.

Vogt, R.L., Hudson, P.J., Orciari, L., Heun, E.M. and Woods, T.C. (1987) Legionnaires' disease and a whirlpool spa. *Annals of Internal Medicine*, **107**(4), 596.

Volk, W.A., Benjamin D.C., Kadner R.J. and Parson J.T. (1991) *Essentials of Medical Microbiology*. Fourth edn. JB Lippincott Company, Philadelphia, USA.

Wang, G. and Doyle, M.P. (1998) Survival of enterohaemmorhagic *Eschericheria coli* 0157:H7 in water. *Journal of Food Protection*, **61**(6), 662–667.

Wang, X., Sturegard, E., Rupar, R., Nilsson, H.-O., Aleljung, P.A., Carlen, B., Willen, R. and Wadstrom, T. (1997) Infection of BALB/cA mice by spiral and coccoid forms of *Helicobacter pylori*. *Journal of Medical Microbiology*, **32**, 3075–3077.

Warren, J.R. and Marshall, B.J. (1984) Unidentified curved bacilli in the stomach of patients with gastritis and peptic ulceration. *Lancet*, **1**(8390), 1311–1315.

Wenz, M., Gorissen, W.M. and Weishammer, S. (2001) Weil's syndrome with bone marrow involvement while collecting walnuts. *Deutsch Medizinische Wochenschrift*, **126**, 1132–1135.

Whitehead, S.E., Allen, K.D., Abernethy, V.E., Feldberg, L. and Ridyard, J.B. (2003) *Mycobacterium malmoense* septic arthritis. *Journal of Infection*, **46**, 60–71.

WHO (1996) *Guidelines for drinking water quality*, 2nd edn, vol.2, *Health Criteria and Other Supporting Information*. WHO, Geneva.

WHO (1986) *Weekly Epidemiological Record*, **61**, 118–120.

WHO (1997) Multi-drug resistant *Salmonella typhimurium*. Fact Sheet No. 139. Available online. http://www.who.int/inf-fs/en/fact139.html.

WHO (1999) Leptospirosis worldwide 1999. *Weekly Epidemiological Record*, 74, 237–244.

WHO (2003) State of the art of new vaccines: research and development. Available on-line http://www.who.int/vaccine_research/documents/new_vaccines/en/index8.html.

WHO (2004a) *Guidelines for drinking-water quality*. 3rd edn, Volume 1, Recommendations. World Health Organization, Geneva, Switzerland.

WHO (2004b) Section V: Categories of waterborne disease organisms. In: *Waterborne zoonoses: Identification, causes and control.* (ed. J.A. Cotruvo, A. Dufour, G. Rees, J. Bartram, R. Carr, D.O. Cliver, G.F. Craun, R. Fayer and V.P.J. Gannon), pp. 210–333. IWA Publishing, London.

WHO (2004c) *Pathogenic mycobacteria in water. A guide to public health consequences, monitoring and management.* (ed. S. Pedley, J. Bartram, G. Rees, A. Dufour and J.A. Cotruvo). IWA Publishing, London.

WHO (2005a) Enterohaemorrhagic *Eshericheria coli* (ECEH) factsheet. http://www.who.int/mediacentre/factsheets/fs125/en/. Accessed 6 July 2005.

WHO (2005b) *Guidelines for safe recreational-water environments*: vol. 2: swimming pools, spas and similar recreational water environments. WHO, Geneva.

WHO (2005c) Flooding and communicable diseases fact sheet. http://www.who.int/hac/techguidance/ems/flood_cds/en/. Accessed 23 June 2005.

WHO (2005d) http://www.who.int/vaccine_research/diseases/shigella/en/. Accessed 6 July 2005.

Wilson, W.H. (1995) Eczema responsive to treatment for *Helicobacter pylori*. *Annals of Allergy, Asthma and Immunology: Official Publication of the American College of Allergy, Asthma and Immunology,* **75**(3), 290.

Winer, J.B., Hughes, R.A.C., Anderson, M.J., Lones, D.M., Kangro, H. and Watkins, R.P.F. (1988) A prospective study of acute idiopathic neuropathy II. Antecedent events. *Journal of Neurology, Neurosurgery and Psychiatry*, **51**, 613–618.

Winthrop, K.L., Abrams, M., Yakrus, M., Schwartz, I., Ely, J., Gillies, D. and Vugia, D.J. (2002) An outbreak of mycobacterial furunculosis associated with footbaths at a nail salon. *New England Journal of Medicine,* **346**(18), 1366–1371.

Wirguin, I., Briani, C., Suturkova-Milosevic, L., Fisher, T., Della-Latta, P., Chalif, P. and Latov, N. (1997) Induction of anti-GM1 ganglioside antibodies by *Campylobacter jejuni* lipopolysaccharides. *Journal of Neuroimmunology,* **78**(1–2), 138–142.

Yabuuchi, E., Wang, L., Arakawa, M. and Yano, I. (1994) Distribution of legionellae in hot spring bath water in Japan. *The Journal of the Japanese Association for Infectious Diseases,* **68**(4), 549–551.

Yamamoto, J., Ishikawa, A., Miyamoto, M., Nomura, T., Uchimura, M. and Koiwai, K. (2001) Outbreak of enterohaemorrhagic *Escherichia coli* O157 mass infection caused by "whole roasted cow". *Japanese Journal of Infectious Diseases,* **54**(2), 88–89.

Yamauchi, T., Yamamoto, S., Fukumoto, M., Oyama, N., Nakano, A., Nakayama, T., Iwasaki, H., Shimizu, H., Tsutani, H., Lee, J.D., Okada, K. and Ueda, T. (1998) Early manifestation of septic shock and disseminated intravascular coagulation complicated by acute myocardial infarction in a patient suspected of having Legionnaires' disease. *The Journal of the Japanese Association for Infectious Diseases,* **72**(3), 286–292.

Yao, T., Matsui, T. and Hiwatashi, N. (2000) Crohn's Disease in Japan. *Diseases of the Colon and Rectum,* **43**, S85–S93.

Yoo, S., Pai, H., Byeon, J. and Lee, B.K. (2002) The incidence and antibiotic resistance patterns of typhoid fever in Korea for recent 10 years. *Annals of Epidemiology,* **12**(7), 24–52.

5

Protozoa and Trematodes

This chapter summarises the evidence for protozoan illnesses acquired through ingestion or inhalation of water or contact with water during water-based recreation. Information on schistosomiasis a disease caused by a parasitic flat worm (trematode) is also presented. The organisms that will be described are: *Cryptosporidium parvum; Giardia duodenalis;* Microsporidia; *Naegleria fowleri and Schistosoma* spp. The following information for each organism is presented: general description, health aspects, evidence for association with recreational waters and a conclusion summarising the weight of evidence.

CRYPTOSPORIDIUM PARVUM

Credibility of association with recreational water: Strongly associated

I Organism

Pathogen

Cryptosporidium parvum

Taxonomy

Cryptosporidium parvum belongs to the phylum Apicomplexa (Sporozoa), class Coccidea and family Cryptosporidiidae. Within the genus *Cryptosporidium* there are ten recognised species (O'Donoghue 1995). The species of concern to humans is *C. parvum*, which has been detected in 152 species of mammals.

Reservoir

C. parvum is an obligate enteric coccidian parasite that infects the gastrointestinal tract of humans and livestock. Oocysts of *Cryptosporidium* are widespread in the environment including lakes and streams. *Cryptosporidium* becomes a problem in surface waters in most areas during spring rains which increase run-off, and many neonate animals are present in the environment to amplify oocyst numbers. Many adult animals continue to produce low levels of oocysts on a regular basis, which enhances the environmental load and serves as a source of infection for neonates (Castro-Hermida 2002). Breakdowns or overloading of public water utilities have resulted in community outbreaks of cryptosporidiosis. It is nearly impossible to determine the origin of many individual cases of cryptosporidiosis. There are many anecdotal reports of the parasite being acquired from public water supplies. Many cases may represent cases of cryptosporidiosis transmitted to humans by companion animals such as kittens and puppies, or by contact with other humans (Tzipori and Ward 2002).

Distribution

Worldwide. Infection and illness caused by *Cryptosporidium* spp. has been reported in more than 40 countries on six continents. Infection is common in developed regions and nearly universal in impoverished areas (Kosek *et al.* 2001).

Characteristics

Oocysts are able to survive for several months in water kept at 4 °C, but at higher temperatures viability decreases more rapidly (Smith and Rose 1990).

Increased rainfall is associated with increased concentrations of oocysts in receiving waters (Atherholt *et al.* 1998). Other factors affecting the presence of oocysts in the water environment are the incidence of infection in the animal or human population, the type of animal waste handling and sewage treatment, and the type of disposal of sewage.

II Health aspects

Primary disease symptoms and sequelae

Cryptosporidiosis is generally a mild self-limiting disease in immunocompetent persons but more serious in the immunocompromised. Infection with *C. parvum* results in severe watery diarrhoea which lasts between several days and two to three weeks in previously healthy persons. Patients may also experience mild abdominal pain and fever. In children from developing countries it has been shown that infection with *C. parvum* predisposes to substantially increased diarrhoeal illnesses (Guerrant *et al.* 2002) and shortfalls in linear growth and weight gain (Checkley *et al.* 1997; Kosek *et al.* 2001). Chan *et al.* (1994) emphasise the lasting consequences where children are infected at an early age. Studies have shown a reduced physical fitness four to six years later associated with early childhood diarrhoea and, specifically with cryptosporidial infections in the first two years of life (Guerrant *et al.* 1999). The fitness deficits alone are comparable with that associated with a 17% reduction in work productivity (Ndamba *et al.* 1993). Work in Brazil has shown that early childhood diarrhoea is associated with long-term cognitive deficits (Guerrant *et al.* 1999) and, more recently, educational performance (Lorntz *et al.* 2000).

Severe diarrhoea is associated with weight loss. Malaise and fever are also common with cryptosporidial infections. Non-gastrointestinal illness, such as cholecystitis, hepatitis and respiratory disease may also occur.

Disease-parasite development and replication is relatively confined to the terminal jejunum and ileum in immunocompetent patients but in immunocompromised patients the entire gastrointestinal tract as well as biliary and pancreatic ducts may become infected (Current and Garcia 1991). Such patients could experience self-limited infection or an acute dehydrating diarrhoeal syndrome (Kosek *et al.* 2001).

While reactive arthritis has been frequently described in association with bacterial pathogens, arthritis linked to parasitic infection has rarely been documented (Sing *et al.* 2003). Reactive arthritis complicating cryptosporidial infection is even rarer; Sing *et al.* (2003) reviews three cases reported by Hay *et al.* (1987); Shepherd *et al.* (1989); Cron and Sherry (1995) and Winchester *et al.* (1987).

cryptosporidiosis was reported amongst swimmers at a swimming pool in Los Angeles, United States (Anonymous 1990). The attack rate of this first outbreak was about 73% and swimmers had been exposed to a single faecal incident. The United States alone had over 170 outbreaks associated with recreational waters in the period 1989–1999 (Anonymous 2000a).

Table 5.1 summarises some recreational water outbreaks documented between 1986 and 2001. These and other published cases linked to recreational waters are described below. Craun *et al.* (1998) have reviewed some of the outbreaks in the United Kingdom and north America. Where information was available they reported attack rates of between 1% and 60% (average 22%), and hospitalisation rates from 1% to 44% (average 13%). There was no correlation between these two figures suggesting that virulence of the organism is not associated with the level of contamination and the distribution.

Table 5.1 Some published cases of cryptosporidiosis outbreaks in recreational waters 1986–2001 (Fayer *et al.* 2000; Rose *et al.* 2002; CDR Weekly website: hpa.org.uk)

Year	Location	Facility	Disinfectant	No. of cases estimated (confirmed)
1986	New Mexico, United States	Lake	None	56
1988	Doncaster, England	Pool	Chlorine	(79)
1988	Los Angeles county, United States	Pool	Chlorine	44 (5)
1990	British Columbia, Canada	Pool	Chlorine	66 (23)
1992	Gloucestershire, England	Pool	Chlorine	(13)
1992	Idaho, United States	Water Slide	Ozone/ Chlorine	500
1992	Oregon, United States	Pool (wave)	Chlorine	(52)
1993	Wisconsin, United States	Pool (motel)	Chlorine	51 (22)
1993	Wisconsin, United States	Pool (motel)	Chlorine	64
1993	Wisconsin, United States	Pool	Chlorine	5
1993	Wisconsin, United States	Pool	Chlorine	54
1994	Missouri, United States	Pool (motel)	Chlorine	101 (26)
1994	New Jersey, United States	Lake	None	2070 (46)
1994	South west England	Pool	Chlorine	14 (8)
1994	Sutherland, Australia	Pool	Chlorine	(70)
1995	Kansas, United States	Pool	*	101 (2)
1995	Georgia, United States	Water Park	Chlorine	2470 (6)
1995	Nebraska, United States	Water Park	*	(14)
1996	Florida, United States	Pool	*	22 (16)
1996	California, United States	Water Park	Chlorine	3000 (29)
1996	Andover, England	Pool	Chlorine	8
1996	Indiana, United States	Lake	None	3

Year	Location	Facility	Disinfectant	No. of cases estimated (confirmed)
1997	England and Wales	River	None	27 (7)
1997	England and Wales	Pool	Ozone/ Chlorine	(9)
1997	Minnesota, United States	Fountain	(Sand Filter)	369 (73)
1997	Queensland, Australia	Pools	*	129
1998	Canberra, Australia	3 Pools	*	(210)
1998	Oregon, United States	Pool	*	51 (8)
1998	New South Wales, Australia	Pools	*	370
1998	Hutt Valley, New Zealand	Pools	*	(171)
1998	Minnesota, United States	Pool	*	(26)
1999	Florida, United States	Interactive water fountain	Chlorine	38 (2)
2000	Ohio, United States	Pool	*	700 (186)
2000	Nebraska, United States	Pool	*	225 (65)
2000	Trent region, England	Pool	Chlorine	41 (41)
2000	London, England	Pool	Chlorine	3 (3)
2001	South west England	Pool	Chlorine	14 (8)
2001	South west England	Stream onto Beach	None	14 (6)

* = data not available

Swimming pools

The source of cryptosporidiosis in swimming pools is generally either sewage or the bathers themselves.

Between August and October 1988, a total of 67 cases of cryptosporidiosis were reported to the Doncaster Royal Infirmary Laboratory in the United Kingdom. An investigation implicated a swimming pool at the local sports centre where oocysts were identified in the pool water. It was shown that effluent was entering from the main sewage into the circulating pool water. An epidemiological investigation confirmed a link between head immersion and illness (Joce et al. 1991).

In 1990 an outbreak of cryptosporidiosis was reported from British Columbia, Canada. A case-control study indicated that transmission occurred in a public children's pool at the local recreation centre and analysis using laboratory-confirmed cases showed that the illnesses were associated with swimming in the children's pool within two weeks prior to the start of the illness. Attack rates ranged from 8% to 78% for various groups of children's pool users (Bell et al. 1993).

In 1992 public health officials in Oregon, United States, identified 55 patients with cryptosporidiosis. A case-control study involving the first 18 case patients showed no association between illness and attendance at a day care centre, drinking municipal water or drinking untreated surface water. However, 9 of the 18 case patients reported swimming at the local wave pool, whereas none of the controls indicated this activity. Of the 18 case patients, 17 were eventually identified as swimming in the same wave pool and it was concluded that the outbreak of cryptosporidiosis was likely to have been caused by exposure to faecally-contaminated wave pool water (McAnulty *et al.* 1994).

In August 1993, a young girl from Wisconsin, United States, was reported to be ill with a laboratory-confirmed *Cryptosporidium* infection and members of her swimming team were also reported to be suffering from severe diarrhoea (Anonymous 1994). Out of 31 people attending the pool who were interviewed 55% reported having watery diarrhoea for two or more days. Of the 17 cases 47% had had watery diarrhoea for more than five days. A second cluster of nine cases was identified later in the month. Seven of the nine reported swimming in a large outdoor pool which was implicated in the outbreak.

An outbreak of gastrointestinal illness was experienced by 61 resort hotel guests during April 1993 in Oshkosh, Wisconsin, United States. Of the guests reporting symptoms, 51 individuals met the case definition for cryptosporidiosis. A case-control study was undertaken among groups who reported illness and among those who stayed at the hotel during the risk period. Swimming in the hotel pool was significantly associated with case status and found to be the only risk factor significantly associated with illness (MacKenzie *et al.* 1995).

From December 1997 to April 1998, 1060 laboratory-confirmed cases of cryptosporidiosis were reported in New South Wales, Australia. In a case-control study it was found that compared with controls, those infected were more likely to be younger (average age 4.2 years) and more likely to report swimming at a public pool or in a dam, river or lake. As only 59% of the cases reported swimming during their exposure periods it was concluded that the remaining cases are likely to have been infected through person-to-person transmission or through other unidentified routes (Puech *et al.* 2001).

Cryptosporidiosis and surface waters

There are a number of reports of people being infected with *Cryptosporidium* spp. after drinking water taken from surface waters but very few published cases of people contracting cryptosporidiosis after swimming in surface waters.

The first reported outbreak in the United States of cryptosporidiosis associated with a recreational lake was reported by Kramer *et al.* (1998). This occurred in the summer of 1994 at a state park in New Jersey. A cohort study was organised with 185 people, 38 of whom had laboratory-confirmed cryptosporidiosis or gastrointestinal illness meeting clinical definitions. Swimming in or exposure to the lake water was strongly associated with illness. The outbreak lasted four weeks and affected an estimated 2070 people. The most likely sources of the outbreak were contaminated rainwater run-off and infected bathers. This investigation highlights the fact that even a large and ongoing epidemic may not be detected for several weeks.

Gallaher *et al.* (1989) report a case-control study of laboratory-confirmed cases of cryptosporidiosis in New Mexico, United States. The study investigated 24 positive stool cases and 46 matched controls. Significant risk factors included swimming in surface water, although this was not the only risk factor. In total, 8 of the 24 cases were exposed to surface water.

Fountains

Between August 7 and 27 1999, 38 people experienced gastrointestinal illnesses following visits to a beachside park in Florida, United States (Anonymous 2000b). The most common symptoms included diarrhoea (97%), abdominal cramps (90%), fever (82%), vomiting (66%) and bloody diarrhoea (13%). *C. parvum* oocysts were identified in two persons' stool samples. All 38 people had entered an interactive water fountain at the beach and all but two had ingested water from it. This fountain used water that recirculated from wet deck/play area flooring into an underground reservoir. This water did not pass through a filtration system but was passed through a hypochlorite tablet chlorination system. However, chlorine levels were not monitored and hypochlorite tablets had not been replaced. The fountain was used by many children of nappy-wearing age. The local health department closed the fountain for over three months while several control measures were employed. A cartridge filtration system was installed and a chlorine monitor put in place to automatically stop the fountain when levels fell beneath 3 ppm. A sign was posted advising visitors to shower before entering the fountain and to avoid drinking the water. Children in nappies/diapers were forbidden from entering the fountain. No further cases were reported.

Several cases of gastroenteritis were identified in visitors to the Minnesota Zoo, United States, in July 1997 (Anonymous 1998). *Cryptosporidium* oocysts were identified in nine out of ten stool specimens submitted by patients. A decorative fountain was implicated as the source. This sprayed jets of water vertically up to approximately 1.8 m. The drained water collected in trenches, passed through a sand filter, was chlorinated and then re-circulated. Water was replaced three times every week but the filter was not flushed. Children were often seen near the fountain on hot days and food was often consumed in its vicinity. In all, 369 cases were identified with 73 laboratory confirmations of *Cryptosporidium*. 95% of all cases were in people under ten years of age. The most common symptoms included diarrhoea (86%), abdominal cramps (78%), vomiting (63%) and bloody diarrhoea (3%). The median incubation after fountain exposure was six days. In addition to fountain exposure, nine cases of cryptosporidiosis were identified among household contacts of case-patients with direct exposure. The source of the outbreak was not identified but contamination by a child wearing a nappy/diaper was suspected. Animals in a petting area approximately 45 m from the fountain tested negative for *Cryptosporidium* spp.

IV Conclusions

Most of the cases of cryptosporidiosis associated with recreational waters have been documented in the United Kingdom or the United States. Faecal accidents are implicated in most of the cases as the cause of the outbreaks, which have primarily occurred in swimming pools, although some cases have been documented from water slides, fountains and water parks. The risk of death and probability of developing long-term sequelae from this infection is low, however the acute illness can be prolonged and moderately severe especially in immunocompromised persons.

Cryptosporidiosis	Epidemiological evidence linking recreational water use with illness	Evidence from outbreak data of illness associated with recreational water	Documented cases of illness associated with recreational water	Documented cases of sequelae (in any situation)
	√	√	√	√

GIARDIA DUODENALIS

Credibility of association with recreational water: Strongly associated

I Organism

Pathogen

Giardiasis is a diarrhoeal illness caused by *Giardia duodenalis* (previously known as *G. lamblia*), a one-celled, microscopic parasite that lives in the intestine of humans and other large mammals.

Taxonomy

The genus *Giardia* belongs to the order Diplomonadida and the family Hexamitidae. There are three known species of *Giardia* – *G. duodenalis* being the only species to infect humans.

Reservoir

Although there are extensive animal reservoirs of *G. duodenalis* it is unclear whether these are significant sources of human disease. Most outbreaks have been linked to consumption of water contaminated by human faeces (Thompson *et al.* 2000).

Distribution

Distribution is worldwide.

Characteristics

G. duodenalis is a binucleated, flagellated protozoan parasite that inhabits the upper small intestine of its vertebrate hosts.

II Health aspects

Primary disease symptoms and sequelae

During the past two decades, *Giardia* has become recognised in many countries as one of the most common causes of waterborne disease (drinking and recreational) in humans.

Infection with *G. duodenalis* begins with asymptomatic cyst passage, acute usually self-limited diarrhoea and a chronic syndrome of diarrhoea, malabsorption, and weight loss. Several strains of *G. duodenalis* have been isolated and described through analysis of their proteins and DNA; type of strain, however, is not consistently associated with disease severity. Different individuals show various degrees of symptoms when infected with the same strain, and the symptoms of an individual may vary during the course of the disease.

Some individuals (less than 4%) remain symptomatic more than two weeks. Symptoms include acute onset of diarrhoea, loose or watery stool, stomach cramps, bloating and upset stomach. These symptoms may lead to weight loss and dehydration. Infections in adults may be asymptomatic. In otherwise healthy persons, symptoms may last between two and six weeks. Occasionally, symptoms may last months to years. In chronic giardiasis the symptoms are recurrent and malabsorption and debilitation may occur. Malabsorption develops in about 10% of chronic cases (Hunter 1998).

About 40% of those who are diagnosed with giardiasis demonstrate disaccharide intolerance during detectable infection and up to six months after the infection can no longer be detected. Lactose intolerance is most frequently observed. Chronic cases of giardiasis in immunodeficient and normal individuals are frequently refractile to drug treatment. In some immune deficient individuals, giardiasis may contribute to a shortening of the life span (Farthing 1994; Lane and Lloyd 2002).

Hill *et al.* (2003) report the development of inflammatory arthritis following enteric infections with *Giardia* spp.

Exposure/mechanisms of infection

The cyst form of the parasite is protected by an outer shell that allows it to survive outside the body in the environment for long periods of time. *Giardia* cysts can survive in the aquatic environments and, if viable, can infect susceptible individuals after oral ingestion of faecally-contaminated food or water. Drinking water, recreational water, food and person-to-person contact have been reported to play a role in the transmission of this parasite (Stuart *et al.* 2003). *Giardia* lives in the intestine of infected humans or animals. Millions of cysts can be released in a bowel movement from an infected human or animal.

The disease mechanism is unknown, with some investigators reporting that the organism produces a toxin while others are unable to confirm its existence. The organism has been demonstrated inside host cells in the duodenum, but most investigators think this is such an infrequent occurrence that it is not responsible for disease symptoms. Mechanical obstruction of the absorptive surface of the intestine has been proposed as a possible pathogenic mechanism, as has a synergistic relationship with some of the intestinal flora.

Disease incidence

G. *duodenalis* is the most frequent protozoan agent of intestinal disease world-wide causing an estimated 2.8×10^8 cases per annum (Lane and Lloyd 2002).

In developed countries, prevalence peaks between the ages of one and four years (Flannagan 1992) and again in the age group 20 to 40 years, due to transmission from children and from travel. In developing countries, the prevalence of giardiasis in patients with diarrhoea is about 20% (Islam 1990). In developed countries the figure varies from 3% (Farthing 1994) to 7% (Quinn 1971).

Incubation period

Incubation is normally between 5 and 25 days. Acute giardiasis develops after an incubation period of between five and six days and usually lasts from one to three weeks (Hunter 1998).

Infectivity

One or more cysts may cause disease. It is estimated that of 100 people ingesting *Giardia* cysts between 5% and 15% will become asymptomatic cyst passers, between 25% and 50% will become symptomatic with an acute diarrhoeal syndrome, and the remaining 35% to 70% will have no trace of the infection (Mandell *et al.* 1995).

Sensitive groups

Giardiasis occurs throughout the population, although the prevalence is higher in children than adults. Chronic symptomatic giardiasis is more common in adults than children (Lane and Lloyd 2002).

Predisposition to giardiasis has been documented in patients with common variable immunodeficiency and in children with x-linked agammaglobulinemia. These patients have symptomatic disease with prolonged diarrhoea, malabsorption and marked changes in bowel biopsy (Lane and Lloyd 2002).

Persons at increased risk of giardiasis include child care workers, children who attend day care centres, international travellers, hikers, campers, swimmers, and others who drink or accidentally swallow water from contaminated sources that is untreated (no heat inactivation, filtration, or chemical disinfection). This disease afflicts many homosexual men, both HIV-positive and HIV-negative individuals.

III Evidence for association of *Giardia* with recreational waters

Giardia has been shown to be transmitted during swimming (Johnson *et al.* 1995) and *Giardia* cysts have been isolated readily from surface water samples (Le Chevallier *et al.* 1991), from water samples taken from coastal beaches (Ho and Tam 1998; Lipp *et al.* 2001), rivers used for recreational activities (Bing-Mu *et al.* 1999) and swimming pools (Fournier *et al.* 2002). Because *Giardia* is known to have a high infectivity and is relatively resistant to disinfection processes the protozoan in recreational waters poses a health risk to users.

Stuart *et al.* (2003) undertook a case-control study in a population in south-west England with a history of diarrhoea and *Giardia* cysts in their stool specimens. None of the participants had travelled outside the United Kingdom in the three-week-period before the onset of diarrhoea. Among other risk factors the study showed an association between giardiasis and swallowing water while swimming. A higher risk of exposure to recreational freshwater was found to be in accordance with other similar studies (Gray and Rouse 1992; Neal and Slack 1997).

In 1984, a case of giardiasis was reported in a child who had participated in an infant swimming class in Washington State, United States (Harter *et al.* 1984). Stool survey of the 70 participants in the class showed 61% prevalence of *Giardia* infection. None of the children present at the pool but not swimming was positive.

In the autumn of 1985, an outbreak of giardiasis occurred among several swimming groups at an indoor pool in north-east New Jersey, United States (Porter *et al.* 1988). Nine clinical cases were identified, eight of these had *Giardia*-positive stool specimens. All were female, seven were over 18 years of age, and two were children. An attack rate of 39% was observed for the group of women who had exposure on one day. These cases had no direct contact with children or other risk factors for acquiring *Giardia*. It was concluded that infection most likely occurred following ingestion of swimming pool water contaminated with *Giardia* cysts. The source was traced to a child who had a faecal accident in the pool on the same day as the women's swimming group. Nine of the 20 members of the child's group were found to have stool samples positive for *Giardia*.

In 1988, an outbreak of giardiasis was associated with a hotel's new water slide pool in Manitoba, Canada (Greensmith *et al.* 1988). Among 107 hotel guests and their visitors surveyed, 29 probable and 30 laboratory-confirmed cases of *Giardia* infection were found. Cases ranged from 3 to 58 years of age. Significant associations were found for staying at the hotel, using the pool's water slide and swallowing pool water. A possible contributing factor was a toddler's wading pool, a potential source of faecal material, to the water slide.

Surveillance data

The greatest number of reports of giardiasis are received during the late summer and early autumn. Because case reports can take one to two months to reach the surveillance centres after onset of illness, this peak reflects increased transmission during the summer months and might reflect the increased use by young children of communal swimming venues – a finding consistent with *Giardia*'s low infectious dose, the high prevalence of children of the age still using nappies/diapers in swimming venues, and *Giardia*'s role as one of the most common causes of recreational water-associated disease outbreaks. Case descriptions of outbreaks of giardiasis associated with recreational waters between 1991 and 1994 in the United States are given in Table 5.2.

Table 5.2 Outbreaks of giardiasis associated with recreational waters 1991–1994 in the United States (Adapted from Furness *et al.* 2000)

Year	Month	Number of cases	Source	Setting
1991	June	14	Swimming pool	Park
1991	July	4	Lake	Campground
1991	July	9	Wading pool	Day care centre
1991	July	7	Wading pool	Day care centre
1993	July	12	Lake	Park
1993	Sept.	43	Lake	Swimming club
1993	Aug.	6	River	River
1994	June	80	Pool	Not specified
1996	June	77	Pool	Community

In 1994, a case-control study was undertaken by Gray *et al.* to determine the risk factors for giardiasis. Giardiasis cases were identified from reports by consultants of the CDC, United States, over a one-year-period and found 74 cases and 108 matched controls. It was concluded that swimming appeared to be an independent risk factor for giardiasis. Travel and type of travel were significant risk factors. Other recreational exposures and ingestion of potentially contaminated water were found not to be significantly related to giardiasis.

In November 1999, epidemiological and microbiological evidence linked the use of a swimming pool to an outbreak of *Giardia* in the west Midlands, United Kingdom. *Giardia* cysts were identified in the water following the report of 16 cases. Between August and November 1999, in East Anglia and Norfolk, United Kingdom, *Cryptosporidium* and *Giardia*-like cysts were identified in filter samples of a swimming pool and 54 cases were identified. A case-control study showed that illness was significantly associated with the implicated swimming pool (Anonymous 2000a).

In Wales, United Kingdom between March and June 2001, 17 cases of *Giardia* were reported from a children's nursery. Pupils, staff, and household contacts of symptomatic individuals were screened. A statistical association for children with water play was found and water play was suspended. Treatment of the microbiologically confirmed source was undertaken. A strong association with water was concluded (Anonymous 2001).

IV Conclusions

Recreational use of water is a proven risk factor for giardiasis. The majority of symptomatic patients of giardiasis will clear their infection after one to several weeks although immunocompromised patients may not recover from giardiasis. The risk of death and the probability of developing sequelae from this infection is low, however the acute illness can be prolonged and moderately severe.

Giardiasis	Epidemiological evidence linking recreational water use with illness	Evidence from outbreak data of illness associated with recreational water	Documented cases of illness associated with recreational water	Documented cases of sequelae (in any situation)
	√	√	√	√

MICROSPORIDIA

Credibility of association with recreational water: Strongly associated

I Organism

Pathogen

Microsporidiosis is caused by microsporidia, a non-taxonomic term to describe a group of protozoa.

Taxonomy

The microsporidia are obligate intercellular spore-forming protozoa belonging to the phylum Microspora (WHO 2004a). This is a large phylum of organisms that include over 700 species which infect all studied insects and animals (James 1997). Microsporidia were once included in the phylum Sporozoa but subsequent research has shown that the microsporidia are a well-defined group with no known relationships with other protists (Dowd 2002). At least six genera of microsporidia are recognised as etiologic agents of disease in humans (Dowd 2002):

(1) *Enterocytozoon bieneusi*
(2) *Encephalitozoon* spp. (*Encephalitozoon intestinalis*), *Encephalitozoon hellem*, and *Enterocytozoon cuniculi*
(3) *Pleistophora*
(4) *Vittaforma cornea*
(5) *Nosema* spp. (*Nosema connori* and *Nosema ocularum*)
(6) *Trachipleistophora hominis*

Human enteropathogenic microsporidia are an important cause of parasitic infections that have emerged in the context of the HIV/AIDS epidemic (James 1997).

Two species are implicated in diarrhoea and other gastrointestinal disease in HIV-infected patients: *Enterocytozoon bieneusi* and *Encephalitozoon intestinalis* (Ferreira *et al.* 2001).

The microsporidia identified in AIDS and other patients are given in Table 5.3.

Table 5.3 Microsporidia identified as human pathogens. The site of infection is denoted by the superscript number (Franzen and Muller 1999; Weiss 2001)

AIDS Patients	*Encephalitozoon[1], Encephalitozoon intestinalis[1], Enterocytozoon cuniculi[1], Enterocytozoon bieneusi[2], Pleistophora* spp.[3], *Nosema ocularum[4], Brachiola, Nosema connori[1], Nosema algerae[4], Vittaforma cornea[4], Microsporidium[1], Microsporidium africanus, Microsporidium ceylonesis*
Other patients	*Encephalitozoon[1], Encephalitozoon hellem[1], Enterocytozoon cuniculi[1], Encephalitozoon intestinalis[1], Enterocytozoon bieneusi[2], Trachipleistophora hominis[3,5], Trachipleistophora anthropopthera[1], Pleistophora* spp.[3], *Brachiola, Brachiola vesicularum, Nosema algerae[4]*

1 = Disseminated; 2 = Small intestine, gall bladder, liver; 3 = Skeletal muscle;
4 = Corneal Stoma; 5 = Nasal sinuses

Reservoir

The environmental sources of microsporidia are poorly characterised. *Encephalitozoonidae* are widely distributed parasites in birds and mammals and the onset of microsporidiosis has been associated with exposure to livestock, fowl and pets (Weiss 2001). Thus encephalitozoonidae infections may be zoonotic, though no direct evidence of this exists.

E. bieneusi have been implicated in water and food transmission routes with spores in water and on undercooked or uncooked food. Final hosts are humans and rhesus monkeys. *E. cuniculi* have similar transmission routes and final hosts include man, pets and animals around the dwelling place (e.g. rabbits, mice, pigs, cows and goats).

Distribution

Distribution is worldwide. Many infections with different species of microsporidia have been reported from all over the world (Franzen and Muller 2001).

Characteristics

Microsporidia form characteristic unicellular spores that are environmentally resistant. *E. cuniculi* spores remain viable for six days in water and four weeks when dry at 22 °C while *N. bombycis* may remain viable for ten years in distilled water (Weiss 2001). Koudela *et al.* (1999) demonstrated that spores remained infective after freezing (down to –70 °C) but lost infectivity in water that reached a temperature of 60 °C at five minutes. Once released into the aquatic environment therefore, these spores may stay viable for some time and so pose a threat of infection for a significant period.

A defining characteristic of all microsporidia is an extrusion apparatus consisting of a polar tube that is attached to the inside of the anterior end of the spore by an anchoring disk and then forms a number of coils around the sporoplasm. A more detailed description of the microbiology and molecular biology of microsporidia are given by Weiss (2001).

Human enteropathogenic microsporidia are closer in size to bacteria (approximately 1 μm to 2 μm in diameter) than to other protozoan parasites such as *Giardia duodenalis* and *Cryptosporidium parvum* (Dowd 2002).

II Health aspects

Primary disease symptoms and sequelae

While infection of the digestive tract is the most common clinical manifestation, infections of the reproductive, respiratory, muscle, excretory and nervous tissue also occur (Weiss 2001). Table 5.4 shows clinical manifestations of human microsporidial infections.

Exposure/mechanisms of infection

The epidemiology of microsporidiosis is largely unknown (Cotte *et al.* 1999). Hutin *et al.* (1998) found in a study of HIV-infected patients that the only factors that were significantly associated with intestinal microsporidiosis were male homosexual preference, swimming in a pool in the previous 12 months and ≤100/mm^3 CD4 lymphocytes. These results, as well as the intestinal localisation of the parasite, suggest a faecal–oral route of transmission (Cotte *et al.* 1999; WHO 2004a).

Co-infection with different microsporidia or other enteric pathogens can occur and microsporidiosis may be linked to travel or residence in the tropics/developing countries (Weiss 2001).

Disease incidence

Prevalence of microsporidia in studies of patients with chronic diarrhoea range from 7% to 50% with the differences in range attributable to factors such as risk factors, diagnostic capability and geographic variation (Slifko *et al.* 2000).

Incubation period

Unknown.

Table 5.4 Clinical manifestations of human microsporidial infections (Adapted from Franzen and Muller 2001)

Species	Clinical manifestation and references to described cases
E. bieneusi	Enteritis, diarrhoea, cholangitis, cholecystitis, pneumonitis, bronchitis, sinusitis, rhinitis
E. intestinalis	Enteritis, diarrhoea, small bowel perforation, cholangitis, cholecystitis, nephritis, urinary tract infection, sinusitis, rhinitis, bronchitis, keratoconjunctivitis, disseminated infection
E. hellem	Keratoconjunctivitis, sinusitis, rhinitis, pneumonitis, nephritis, ureteritis, prostatitis, urethritis, cystitis, disseminated infection
E. cuniculi	Hepatitis, peritonitis, encephalitis, intestinal infection, urinary tract infection, keratoconjunctivitis, sinusitis, rhinitis, disseminated infection (Terada *et al.* 1987; Zender *et al.* 1989)
Encephalitozoon spp.	Cutaneous infection, hepatic failure, bone infection (Matsubayashi *et al.* 1959; Bergquist *et al.* 1984; Yachnis *et al.* 1996)
Trachipleistophtera	Myositis, keratoconjunctivitis, sinusitis, rhinitis
T. anthropophthera	Encephalitis, myositis, disseminated infection (Yachnis *et al.* 1996)
Pleistophora spp.	Myositis (Ledford *et al.* 1985; Chupp *et al.* 1993; Field *et al.* 1996)
Vittaforma corneae	Keratitis, urinary tract infection
Nosema ocularum	Keratoconjunctivits
N. connori	Disseminated infection
Brachiola vesicularum	Mysositis
B. algerae	Keratoconjunctivits
Microsporidium africanum	Corneal ulcer
M. ceylonensis	Corneal ulcer

Infectivity

Very low infective doses are suspected to be necessary for infection (Dowd 2002; WHO 2004a). Microsporidial spores are stable in the environment and remain infective for days to weeks outside their hosts.

Sensitive groups

Human enteropathogenic microsporidia cause chronic diarrhoea and wasting in HIV-infected individuals. Immunocompromised patients are most at risk.

III Evidence for association of microsporidiosis with recreational waters

The presence of microsporidia in recreational water has not been investigated in detail to date although it has been proposed that recreational water contact may be an independent risk factor for intestinal microsporidiosis (Fournier *et al.* 2002). The biological features of microsporidia that favour waterborne transmission are outlined in Table 5.5.

Hutin *et al.* (1998) showed a strong link between occurrence of intestinal microsporidiosis and swimming in a pool within the previous 12 months (43% of case-patients reported this behaviour). This highlights the risk posed by microsporidia in recreational waters. Another preliminary report suggested swimming in a freshwater body was associated with intestinal microsporidiosis in HIV patients (Watson *et al.* 1996). Risk factors identified included swimming in rivers, ponds and lakes and drinking unfiltered tap water.

In 1997 Hutin *et al.* (1998) conducted a case-control study with HIV-infected patients which showed that the only two factors associated with the intestinal microsporidiosis were swimming in a pool and homosexuality. This suggests that transmission is via the faecal–oral route and possibly through contaminated water.

Several studies have identified this pathogen in surface waters. Arcay (2000) has identified microsporidia in an array of river and lakewaters in Venezuela. Fournier *et al.* (2000) identified the presence of *E. bieneusi* from the River Seine in France from 25 samples taken over a one-year-period. Dowd *et al.* (1998) identified microsporidia from a range of water types in the United States. The presence of *E. intestinalis* was confirmed in surface water and groundwater and *E. bieneusi* was identified in surface water.

Table 5.5 The biological features of microsporidia that favour waterborne transmission (Adapted from Franzen and Muller 1999)

Biological feature	Characteristic of microsporidia
Large number of infected host	The number of spores released during infection is not known exactly but is probably large
Lack of host specificity	Reported in a variety of hosts
Robust nature of spores	At 4 °C organisms can survive in water for more than one year
Small size	The size of human microsporidia spores are 1.0 –3.0 μm x 1.5 – 4.0 μm
Low infectious dose	100 spores cause infection in athymic mice

Microsporidia are of concern in recreational water as the spores of some varieties (e.g. *E. cuniculi*) can contaminate the environment via urine as well as faeces (Slifko *et al.* 2000).

Fournier *et al.* (2002) conducted a one-year-study of microsporidia occurrence in six different swimming pools in Paris, France – two were pools used by babies, two used by children, one used by adults and one hot tub used by homosexual men in a private club. Of the 48 samples analysed, one proved positive for microsporidia (from one of the children's pool), one for *Cryptosporidia* and none for *Giardia*. The positive detection of microsporidia was thought to be that of *E. shubergi*, a microsporidia usually found in invertebrates suggesting insect contamination of the pool. The good quality of the pool water reflects on the following procedures:

- The sourcing of pool water from public supply which is already disinfected
- The pools' utilisation of a combination of filtration and disinfection system using either chlorine, bromide or ozone.

The study concluded that swimming pools are rarely contaminated with microsporidia and the risk of contamination through swimming pools is limited.

A presumed waterborne outbreak of microsporidiosis was reported by Cotte *et al.* (1999). In the summer of 1995, 200 people (82% of which were immunocompromised) suffered a waterborne outbreak of microsporidiosis with no evidence of faecal contamination. These patients lived preferentially in an area corresponding to one of the three water distribution systems of Lyon, France suggesting contaminated water. Unfortunately this was a retrospective study and it was therefore not possible to sample the water distribution system for the presence of microsporidia. Factors that may have contributed to contamination include pumping of surface water directly from a recreational area that is mainly frequented by swimmers in summer. Treatment of this water was by flocculation, ozoflotation and filtration instead of by chlorination as at the other two treatment facilities.

Diatomeaceous earth filters used in swimming pools will not filter out microsporidia spores so treatments such as chlorination or ozone are the only possible prevention methods (Hutin *et al.* 1998). Limited work has suggested microsporidia are susceptible to achievable chlorine concentration versus time values (Mota *et al.* 2000). Dowd *et al.* (1998) have confirmed the presence of *E. intestinalis* and *Vittaforma cornea* in tertiary sewage effluent surface water suggesting that microsporidia can survive the wastewater process, including mixed medium filtration and chlorination.

Huffman *et al.* (2002) have shown that UV light at low and medium-pressure can lead to inactivation of >3.6 $\log_{10}$ of *E. intestinalis* at a dose of 6 mJ/cm^2.

Hence UV light at dosages utilised for drinking water treatment is capable of achieving high levels of inactivation of at least certain microsporidia.

IV Conclusions

Although microsporidia are currently not common causes of recreational waterborne disease, their role as emerging pathogens is being increasingly recognised. Their small size makes them difficult to remove by conventional water filtration techniques and it is thought that, like *Cryptosporidium* they may show increased resistance to chlorine disinfection. Illness is generally reported in immunocompromised individuals although some infections in immunocompetent individuals have been reported.

Microspoidiosis	Epidemiological evidence linking recreational water use with illness	Evidence from outbreak data of illness associated with recreational water	Documented cases of illness associated with recreational water	Documented cases of sequelae (in any situation)
	√	√	√	√

NAEGLERIA FOWLERI

Credibility of association with recreational water: Strongly associated

I Organism

Pathogen

Naegleria fowleri.

Taxonomy

The genus *Naegleria* belongs to the Order Schizopyrenida, Family Vahlkamphidae. There are six species in the genus. *N. fowleri* is the primary human pathogen, the disease is known as primary amoebic meningoencephalitis (PAM) and is almost always fatal but uncommon.

Reservoir

N. fowleri is a free-living, thermophilic amoeba that grows well in tropical and subtropical climates, where water temperatures exceed 25–30 °C (WHO 2004a). In colder climates *N. fowleri* encysts at the bottom of lakes, rivers and swimming pools where it may persist in the sediments.

    N. fowleri has been isolated from the thermal discharges of power plants, hot springs, sewage and even from the nasal passages of healthy persons (Martinez and Visvesvara 1991).

Distribution

N. fowleri is found worldwide in freshwater and soil. Most of the reports of PAM have been from developed rather than developing nations. This is probably because of greater awareness of the infection rather than greater incidence. Cases have been reported from Belgium, United Kingdom, India, Ireland, New Zealand, Nigeria, Panama, Puerto Rico, Uganda and Venezuela (De Jonckheere 1987; Anonymous 1992; Kilvington and Beeching 1995).

Characteristics

These are free-living amoeba which normally live as phagotrophs in aquatic habitats where they feed on bacteria, but they are opportunistic pathogens. The life cycle consists of a feeding trophozoite or amoeba, a resting cyst and a transient flagellate.

II Health aspects

Primary disease symptoms and sequelae

Onset of PAM is abrupt, with rapidly progressive headaches, fever, nausea, vomiting, pharyngitis and nasal obstruction or discharge (Martinez 1993). Convulsions may occur together with lethargy, confusion and a stiff neck. Eventually the patient falls into a coma and death usually occurs within 1 to 14 days. Other symptoms include abnormalities of taste and smell; seizures; cerebellar ataxia; nuchal rigidity; photophobia; palsies of the third, fourth and sixth cranial nerves; and increased intracranial pressure. Cardiac abnormalities may also occur. Healthy people may experience subclinical infections where the protozoa colonise the nose and throat.

Exposure/mechanisms of infection

The invasive stage of *N. fowleri* is the amoeba. Infection occurs by intranasal absorption of amoebae in freshwater when water is forcefully inhaled or splashed onto the olfactory epithelium, for example from diving, swimming underwater or jumping. Amoebae enter the nasal mucosa, cribriform plate and olfactory bulbs of the brain. The amoebae then spread to other regions of the brain where they cause inflammation and destruction of the brain tissue and penetrate the central nervous system. Water is the only known source of infection (WHO 2004a).

No figures on the incidence of subclinical infections were found in the literature. One study by Sadaka *et al.* (1994) took samples from different water sources in Alexandria, Egypt and from nasal passages of 500 healthy children inhabiting areas nearby. These sources were examined for the presence of amoebae. The samples were cultured and amoebae were isolated and identified. Nine species, *N. gruberi, N. fowleri, Acanthamoeba rhysodes, A. glebae, A. culbertsoni, A. astronyxis, A. palestinensis, Vahlkampfia avara* and *V. inornata* were isolated from the water of canals and drains. *N. gruberi* and *A. rhysodes* were found in the nasal passages of six healthy children living near the contaminated canals. No amoebae were encountered in the drinking water, swimming pools, sea and lake water included in this study (Martinez and Janitschke 1985).

Disease incidence

PAM is rare in occurrence. According to the CDC, there is an average of one to three infections in the United States each year (Levy *et al.* 1998). Australia, Czechoslovakia and the United States account for 75% of all reported cases of the disease (John 1982). Martinez and Visvesvara (1997) estimated that 179 cases had been reported up to 1997 and of these 81 were in the United States.

Incubation period

There is typically a two-to-seven day incubation period before symptoms of PAM appear (Health Canada 2001).

Infectivity

Not known.

Sensitive groups

No predisposing factors are necessary for human infections to occur (Martinez and Visvesvara 1991) and infection typically occurs in healthy children or young adults with a recent history of swimming or practising water sports in freshwater, heated swimming pools or artificial lakes. Cases have also been reported in persons having no contact with water but contact with mud (Lawande *et al.* 1979).

III Evidence for association of *Naegleria fowleri* with recreational water use

Several hundred cases of disease have been reported and *N. fowleri* has been isolated from recreational waters on many occasions throughout the world. Pernin and Riany (1978) report a study which found that 90% of 44 water samples taken in nine swimming pools in Lyon, France, contained amoebae. The majority of the isolates belonged to genus *Acanthamoeba* and *Hartmannella*. However, *Naegleria* was isolated directly from one of the pools on one occasion.

Wellings *et al.* (1977) found over 60% of Florida lakes were positive for *N. fowleri*.

N. fowleri was isolated from water during a routine inspection of a swimming pool in Prague, Czech Republic in December 1977. This swimming pool was identified as a source of the infectious agent between the years 1962 and 1965, when a large outbreak of PAM occurred involving 19 cases (Kadlec *et al.* 1978). Two strains of *N. fowleri*, pathogenic for white mice after intracerebral and intranasal inoculation, were isolated from water in outlet troughs. Additional strains were then isolated from various places, particularly from a cavity in the damaged wall of the pool. Epidemiological investigations did not reveal any new case of PAM in relation to the occurrence of pathogenic *N. fowleri* in the swimming pool (Kadlec *et al.* 1978).

De Jonckheere (1971) examined one outdoor and 15 indoor swimming pools in Belgium for the presence of amoebae. Of the isolates made from 13 pools, 43.6% belonged to the genus *Acanthamoeba*. The genus *Naegleria* accounted for 7.3% of the isolates, but *N. fowleri* was not recovered from any of the samples.

Gogate and Deodhar (1985) report a study of 12 swimming pools, six small ponds and three lakes in Bombay, India. *N. fowleri* was isolated from one swimming pool sample.

Rivera *et al.* (1990) took seven water samples from three thermal water bathing resorts in Tecozautla, Hidalgo, Mexico and analysed them during December 1984. The group isolated 33 strains of free-living amoebae belonging to the genera *Naegleria, Acanthamoeba*, and *Willaerti.* Of these, 20 of the strains belonged to the *Naegleria* genus, and of these 16 were classified as *Naegleria* spp., and two were classified as *N. lovaniensis*. Two pathogenic strains of the species *N. australiensis* and *N. lovaniensis* were found which may be considered good indicator organisms for the presence of *N. fowleri*.

Rivera *et al.* (1983; 1993) reports a survey of pathogenic and free-living amoebae in swimming pool waters in Mexico City. Among the organisms isolated, those which have public health importance were *N. fowleri* and *A. castellanii*. Amoebae of the genera *Acanthamoeba, Naegleria*, and *Vahlkampfia* were recovered in their cystic stage. Amoebae were concentrated through filtration procedures and subsequently cultured. Most commonly found were amoebae of the species *N. gruberi* (59.02%), *N. fowleri* (16.77%), and *A. castellanii* (7.64%). All isolated strains of *N. fowleri* and *A. castellanii* were thermophilic at 45 °C and 40 °C respectively, and also pathogenic when inoculated into white mice. Indoor swimming pools with an inner side garden were more likely to be contaminated. It was also shown that the residual chlorine values of between 0.50 mg/litre and 1.5 mg/litre, are not adequate for elimination of amoebae.

The majority of published cases of infections with *N. fowleri* are in individuals who have had a recent history of swimming in freshwater during hot weather.

The first four human cases of fatal PAM caused by free-living amoebas were reported by Fowler and Carter (1965). Several studies since have identified the *Naegleria* amoeba as a cause of illness following the use of recreational waters. In Usti, Czech Republic, 16 cases were associated with a public swimming pool (Cerva and Novak 1968).

Duma *et al.* (1971) report 16 cases of PAM associated with individuals swimming in a lake in Virginia, United States.

The first documented case of PAM caused by *N. fowleri* in recreational water in Mexico was in 1978 and reported by Valenzuela *et al.* (1984). A 16-year-old male from Mexicali in the state of Baja California was admitted to hospital in August 1978, seven days after sustaining moderate head trauma while swimming in a shallow, stagnant irrigation ditch on a hot summer day. He developed an acute illness with severe headache, fever and convulsions rapidly progressing into a comatose state. Actively moving trophozoites were observed in his spinal fluid on admission to hospital. The patient died on the third day of symptoms. Post-mortem examination revealed a meningoencephalitis with extensive destruction, haemorrhage and numerous parasites involving structures of the posterior fossa. Immunoperoxidase strains of trophozoites in meningeal and cerebellar tissue were positive for *N. fowleri*.

Rodriguez *et al.* (1998) report the case of a previously healthy 16-year-old male in Argentina who, following immersion in a water tank, was admitted to hospital because of meningeal irritation that progressed to coma and death within days; autopsy revealed PAM by *N. fowleri*.

Lares-Villa *et al.* (1993) describe an outbreak of PAM affecting five individuals in Mexico who had been swimming in the same artificial canal during August and September 1990. All five died.

Three cases of PAM were reported in Britain by Cain *et al.* (1981). In one case a young girl died from PAM after swimming in a thermal spa pool in Bath, United Kingdom in 1978.

DeNapoli *et al.* (1996) report a case of a 13-year-old boy who had been swimming in the Rio Grande, United States, became infected by *N. fowleri* and subsequently developed PAM. Death occurred 36 hours after admission to hospital. It was reported that the Rio Grande is highly polluted with faecal waste and industrial chemicals. The 13-year-old patient swam regularly in the Rio Grande as well as in an adjacent holding pond.

In Thailand, PAM was first reported in 1982. Between 1982 and 1989, five cases were reported (Table 5.6). The first reported case was in a five-year old boy with a history of swimming in a pond along a rice field. He died three days after admission to hospital (Jariya *et al.* 1983).

Another case was a four-and-a-half-year-old girl who had swum in a water supply canal in Bang Kam with her father almost every day for two weeks prior to her illness. None of the other children who had been swimming contracted the disease although the organism was detected in the water source. The girl died on the fifth day of her illness (Sirinavin *et al.* 1989).

Table 5.6 Cases of primary ameobic meningoencephalitis in Thailand, 1982–1989 (Adapted from Sirinavin *et al.* 1989)

Date of disease	Age of patient (years)	Sex
September 1982	5	Male
March 1986	8 and 12	Male
April 1986	17	Male
April 1986	14	Male
May 1987	4	Female

Surveillance data

Outbreaks of disease caused by *N. fowleri* in recreational waters are recorded in the United States by CDC. Table 5.7 shows the cases of PAM from *N. fowleri* in recreational waters recorded in the United States between 1991 and 2000. Eight cases were reported in the United States in 2002 (Yoder *et al.* 2004).

Table 5.7 Cases of primary amoebic meningoencephalitis caused by *N. fowleri* in recreational waters recorded in the United States, 1991–2000 (Anonymous 1992; Kramer *et al.* 1996; Levy *et al.* 1998; Barwick *et al.* 2000; Lee *et al.* 2002)

Year	Month	Source	Number of cases and outcome
1991	October	Hot spring in a recreational area	1 – fatal
1991	August	Falling into a puddle face down after a fight in a rural area	1 – fatal
1991	September	Stream in a rural area	1 – fatal
1991	September	Freshwater pond in a swimming area	1 – fatal
1991	September	Lake in a swimming area	1 – fatal
1991	July	Lake in a swimming area	1 – fatal
1994	July	Pond/river in rural area	1 – fatal
1995	Not specified	Shallow lake, river pond and canal	6 – all fatal
1998	August	Lake	1 – fatal
1998	August	Stream – drainage canal	1 – fatal
1998	August	River	1 – fatal
1998	July	Lake	1 – fatal
1999	October	Pond	1 – fatal
2000	April	Mudhole	1 – fatal
2000	Not reported	Not reported – person fell from jet ski into water and was infected	1 – fatal
2000	July	Lake	1 – fatal

IV Conclusions

Credibility of association of *N. fowleri* with recreational waters is strong. *N. fowleri* has been shown to colonise warm freshwater habitats, such as swimming pools and natural hot springs and there is a high risk of death in infected persons. The acute illness is severe with symptoms lasting more than seven days and death always occuring.

PAM from *N. fowleri*	Epidemiological evidence linking recreational water use with illness	Evidence from outbreak data of illness associated with recreational water	Documented cases of illness associated with recreational water	Documented cases of sequelae (in any situation)
	√	√	√	√

TREMATODE WORM

Credibility of association with recreational water: Strongly associated

I Organism

Pathogen

Schistosomes.

Taxonomy

The human schistosomes belong to the Family Schistosomatoidea, suborder Strigeata. There are five species which are responsible for the majority of disease. These are: *Schistosoma haematobium, S. mansoni, S. japonicum, S. intercalatum* and *S. mekongi*. They differ from other trematodes in that the adults are diecious, parasitise blood vessels, lack a muscular pharynx, produce non-operculate eggs and the circaria invades the host percutaneously.

Reservoir

Schistosomiasis is caused by digenetic blood trematodes. The reservoir for *S. japonicum* is animals, such as water buffalo, pigs and cattle (McGarvey *et al.* 1999).

Distribution

The disease is found worldwide particularly in:
- Africa: southern Africa, sub-Saharan Africa, Lake Malawi, the Nile River valley in Egypt
- South America: including Brazil, Suriname, Venezuela
- Caribbean: Antigua, Dominican Republic, Guadeloupe, Martinique, Montserrat, Saint Lucia (risk is low)
- The Middle East: Iran, Iraq, Saudi Arabia, Syrian Arab Republic, Yemen
- Southern China
- Southeast Asia: Philippines, Laos, Cambodia, Japan, central Indonesia, Mekong delta.

     Cases have also been reported from Europe and the United States.

Characteristics

The snail hosts require freshwater. Alkaline rather than acidic freshwater is preferable since the snails require calcium for their shells. Water temperatures above 20 °C but less than 39 °C are optimum as are areas where plants that the snails feed on are well exposed to sunlight. The snails survive well in slow moving and muddy waters (Hunter 1998).

II Health aspects

Primary disease symptoms and sequelae

Awareness of the disease dates back to the 19th century when the physician Daijiro Fujii described the disease in peasants in the Katayama District of Japan (Savioli *et al.* 1997). There are two forms of acute disease: schistosome dermatitis and Katamaya fever. Schistosome dermatitis is due to the penetration of free-swimming cercariae through the skin (McKerrow and Salter 2002). Symptoms depend upon the infecting species and the worm load. Acute effects are not usually seen in persons living in endemic areas unless they are exposed to a massive infection which may occur, for example, after flooding.

Symptoms usually begin with dermatitis with slight exanthema and itch when the worm penetrates the skin (known as swimmers itch). Dermatitis usually disappears within a week and a cough develops if the worm enters the lungs. This is accompanied by a mild fever and dullness. About one fifth of patients develop anaemia (Hunter 1998).

After a period of approximately one month, the acute phase of the disease may begin with a high fever and rigors (Katayama fever). There is considerable inflammation of the liver and other organs resulting in daily fever, abdominal pain and enlarged and tender spleen and liver. Discharge of eggs into the intestinal canal is accompanied by dysentry or diarrhoea. These symptoms characterise intestinal schistosomiasis (Hunter 1998).

Katamaya fever typically occurs four to six weeks after infection and is usually due to *S. japonicum, S. mansoni* and rarely *S. haematobium*. Katamaya fever can result in death but is not common. Central nervous system schistosomiasis is a rare complication of *S. japonicum* infection (Hunter 1998).

Most persons with schistosomiasis have a moderate to low worm load, and may not show any specific symptoms. However, in patients with a heavy worm load delayed effects arise. These depend upon the organ affected.

Bladder and kidney disease may result from infection with *S. haematobium* which stays in the veins of the genitourinary system. Intestinal and hepatic disease is caused by the other species which enter the mesenteric veins (Hunter 1998).

Hepatosplenic schistosomiasis is characterised by hardness in the liver and liver cirrhosis in severe cases. The spleen becomes enlarged and the abdominal collateral veins dilated. Osesphagogastric varices are seen in advanced cases, and sudden death may occur if these bleed, although they are associated with low mortality. The final stage of hepatosplenic schistosomiasis is the development of decompensated liver disease (Mandell *et al.* 1995). In *S. japonica* embolism of eggs may cause headaches, seizures, paraesthesia and poor vision (Bissessur and Minderhoud 1985). Hepatic coma may occur as a complication.

Fatigue, palpitations, exertional dyspnoea and cough are symptoms of *S. mansoni* infections.

In urinary schistsomiasis ulcers of the bladder mucosa occur causing pain. In extreme cases hydronephrosis may result from obstruction of the urinary tract, causing renal parenchymal dysfunction. Complications resulting in kidney failure may occur if bacteria such as *E. coli*, *Salmonella* spp, *Pseudomonas* spp or *Klebsiella* spp are also present.

There is overwhelming evidence for the association of bladder cancer and *S. haematobium* infections (IARC Working Group on the Evaluation of Carcinogenic Risks to Humans 1994).

Gynaecological organs may also be affected by *S. haematobium* infections. Female genital schistosomiasis may be an important risk factor for transmission of HIV (Feldmeier *et al.* 1995) and there is some published evidence for an association between genital ulcers due to *S. haematobium* infection and HIV infection in women (Poggensee and Feldmeier 2001).

Exposure/mechanism of infection

The main host of all species (except *S. mekongi*) causing schistosomiasis is man. Eggs are passed in the urine or faeces. When the eggs come into contact with freshwater they hatch, releasing the first larval stage (a miracidium) which then penetrates the body of an intermediate host - a freshwater snail. Within the snail the miracidium multiply to form sporocysts. After four to six weeks these are released from the snail as free-swimming cercariae which must penetrate the skin of a host within 72 hours if they are to survive. In order to be infected therefore an individual (the host) must be in contact with water. Whilst penetrating the host they lose their tails and become schistosomula, which then travel to the lungs or liver where they mature and mate. Once they are mature they migrate through the venous system to another site in the body where they remain for five to ten years. The site depends on the species - *S. haematobium* remains in the veins of the bladder; other species remain in the mesenteric vein (Hunter 1998).

Disease incidence

Data (van der Werf *et al.* 2003) indicate that, in terms of morbidity and mortality, schistosomiasis, represents an even greater disease burden than previously appreciated.

WHO estimate that over 200 million people in 74 countries and territories of the world are affected by schistosomiasis and between 500 and 600 million are at risk (WHO 2004b).

Most cases, and all of the most severely affected, are now concentrated in Africa. A number of endemic countries such as Brazil, China, the Philippines and Egypt have been able to sustain national control programmes for a prolonged period, while others, such as Venezuela, Saudi Arabia, Tunisia and Morocco, are nearing eradication or have already achieved this goal (WHO 2004b).

Globally, about 120 million of the 200 million infected people are estimated to be symptomatic, and 20 million are thought to suffer severe consequences of the infection. Yearly, 20,000 deaths are estimated to be associated with schistosomiasis. This mortality is mostly due to bladder cancer or renal failure associated with urinary schistosomiasis and to liver fibrosis and portal hypertension associated with intestinal schistosomiasis (WHO 2004b).

Incubation period

Schistosome dermatitis begins 24 hours after penetration of the cercariae. The next clinical phase (Katayama fever) begins between four and eight weeks later (Mandell *et al.* 1995).

Infectivity

Prevalence and degree of morbidity have been shown to correlate well with the worm burden as estimated by faecal or urinary egg counts (Mandell *et al.* 1995).

Sensitive groups

None. Schistosomiasis can affect all groups.

III Evidence for association with recreational waters

There are many published cases of schistosomiasis contracted through swimming or recreational use of water from throughout the world. Human infections depend on the presence of intermediate snail hosts in bodies of water which may be contaminated with human faeces and excreta. Transmission is influenced by human water contact activities, patterns and duration. Upatham (1976) reported that *S. mansoni* cercariae (in St. Lucia) were carried downstream as far as 195 m in running water habitats. Radke *et al.* (1961) showed that mice could be infected 600 m downstream from the point of *S. mansoni* cercarial released under field conditions. These data showed that geographic characteristics such as water flow along rivers and streams might be important in allowing infection at a contact site away from infected snail colonies.

Ndyomugyenyi and Minjas (2001) looked at prevalence of urinary schistosomiasis in school children in Kinondoni district of Dar-es-Salaam city, Tanzania. Recreational activities such as bathing, swimming and playing in the water were the most frequent activities attracting children to water bodies and carried the highest risks of infection with *S. haematobium*. Boys were more likely to be carrying the infection than girls and the age group 10–14 years had higher prevalence and intensities of infection than those in the younger or older age-group studied.

Ofoezie *et al.* (1998) found similar patterns in children in Nigeria. Those in the 10–14 year age group were more likely to be infected with the schistosomiasis. Most water contacts were of either a recreational (swimming, bathing) or economic (fishing) nature.

Useh and Ejezie (1999) looked at water-contact patterns of 2136 residents of Admin community in Nigeria at four streams between February 1993 and January 1994. Urine samples collected from those observed were used to estimate the prevalence and intensity of *S. haematobium* infection. Infection was detected in 50.4% of the subjects, with peak prevalence among those aged 10–14 years. It was found that intensity of infection was more closely correlated with the number of water contacts than with the total duration of the exposure.

Canoeing in certain South African waters is considered to be a high-risk activity with regard to schistosomiasis, gastroenteritis and possibly hepatitis. In a cross-sectional study, a serosurvey was conducted amongst canoeists to ascertain whether or not they had a higher seroprevalence to HAV, Norovirus and *Schistosoma* spp. than non-canoeists. In comparing the two groups, a significant association could not be demonstrated between canoeing and antibody response to HAV and norovirus (P-values for age-adjusted chi^2 were 0.083 and 0.219 respectively), but a significant association was demonstrated between canoeing and the antibody response to *Schistosoma* spp. (P < 0.001; age-adjusted) (Taylor *et al.* 1995).

A study was carried out by Jeans and Schwellnus (1994) to determine the risk of schistosomiasis in triathletes in Zimbabwe. The prevalence of schistosomiasis in 30 triathletes (24 males, six females) was compared with that in 24 non-triathlete controls after the 1989/1990 triathlon season. All the subjects found to be infected were then treated with praziquantel (40 mg/kg). The seasonal incidence of schistosomiasis in triathletes was then determined in a prospective study during the 1990/1991 season. There was a significantly (P < 0.05) higher prevalence of schistosomiasis among the triathletes (80%) than among the controls (38%). The seasonal incidence of schistosomiasis was 64%. The study concluded that exposure of triathletes to fresh-water dam swimming in Zimbabwe poses a significant risk for the development of schistosomiasis.

In 1992 two United States Peace Corps volunteers developed central nervous system schistosomiasis due to infection with *S. haematobium* following recreational water exposure at Cape Maclear on Lake Malawi. Schistosome-infected *Bulinus globosus*, the snail vector of *S. haematobium* in Malawi, were found at Cape Maclear and other locations along the lakeshore (Cetron *et al.* 1996).

Kloos *et al.* (1983) studied three cohorts of male students from an Egyptian village aged 5–16 during a two-year period. Twelve types of water contact activities were studied and it was concluded that swimming and playing resulted in more frequent and intensive contact with potentially infected water and in more pollution of snail habitats with schistosome eggs than any other type of activity.

Many cases of schistosomiasis in Europe are imported. Corachán *et al.* (1997) report clinical and epidemiological data from 80 Spanish travellers to Mali. A quarter of them showed symptoms related to the genital tract. In some groups, 45% of travellers that had swum, contracted the infection. The most prevalent species diagnosed was *S. haematobium* and ten travellers had mixed infections.

In October 1982 a man from Colorado, United States who had returned from a rafting trip in Ethiopia suffered a low grade fever and myalgia which he did not seek medical help for despite the symptoms persisting. However, in February 1983 he was notified of a case of schistosomiasis that had been diagnosed in a fellow rafter. Stool examination revealed eggs of *S. mansoni*, and his serum was tested positive by the indirect immunofluorescent test for schistosomiasis. It was subsequently revealed that three tour guides had *S. mansoni* diagnosed and 39% of the participants were also infected. No specific site of exposure could be identified. Most participants took few or no precautions other than towelling-off, despite being aware of the risk of acquiring schistosomiasis. However, those who towel-dried most of the time after water exposure had a significantly reduced likelihood of infection; eight of 11 of the non-infected and one of seven of the ill towel-dried after water exposure during the last third of either trip (P = 0.02) (Anonymous 1983).

Surveillance data from the US CDC did not reveal large numbers of cases – in 1996 *Schistosoma* spp were identified as the etiologic agent of two outbreaks (affecting 71 and 50 people respectively) of swimmers itch in 1997 in Oregon, United States. Both outbreaks were from a lake at a beach area (Levy *et al.* 1998).

An estimated 127 persons were affected in eight outbreaks of dermatitis associated with pools, hot tubs, springs or lakes in Oregon, United States. *S. spindale* was the presumed etiologic agent of one of the outbreaks of swimmers itch because the clinical signs were consistent with cercarial dermatitis (Barwick *et al.* 2000).

IV Conclusions

Published cases and epidemiological studies show a clear association of schistosomiasis with recreational use of freshwater around the world. In some cases serious pathology associated with infection by *Schistosoma* spp. occurs and can lead to long-term health issues. Surveillance for schistosomiasis is currently poor, inferring that many more cases associated with recreational waters occur but are not published. Evidence shows that exposure to schistosomes is difficult to avoid but it has been shown that towel-drying after exposure to infested water can markedly reduce the risk of infection.

Schistosomiasis	Epidemiological evidence linking recreational water use with illness	Evidence from surveillance data of illness associated with recreational water	Documented cases of illness associated with recreational water	Documented cases of sequelae (in any situation)
	√	√	√	√

REFERENCES

Anonymous (1983) Schistosomiasis among river rafters in Ethiopia. *MMWR,* **32**(44), 585–586.

Anonymous (1990) Epidemiologic notes and reports swimming associated cryptosporidiosis – Los Angeles County. *MMWR,* **39**(20), 343–345.

Anonymous (1992) Primary amoebic meningoencephalitis – North Carolina, 1991. *MMWR,* **41**(25), 437–440.

Anonymous (1994) *Cryptosporidium* infections associated with swimming pools – Dane County, Wisconsin. *MMWR,* **43**(31), 561–563.

Anonymous (1998) Outbreak of cryptosporidiosis associated with a water sprinkler fountain, Minnesota. *MMWR,* **47**(40), 856–860.

Anonymous (2000a) Surveillance of waterborne diseases and water quality: July to December 1999. *Communicable Disease Report,* **10**(7), 65–67.

Anonymous (2000b) Outbreak of gastroenteritis associated with an interactive water fountain at a beachside park, Florida, 1999. *MMWR,* **49**(25), 565–568.

Anonymous (2001) Surveillance of waterborne disease and water quality: January to June 2001, and summary of 2000. *CDR Weekly,* 8 November, 8.

Anonymous (2004) Cryptosporidium infection.
http://www.cdc.gov/ncidod/dpd/parasites/cryptosporidiosis/factsht_cryptosporidiosis.htm

Arcay, L. (2000) Human microsporidiosis. *Investigacion Clinica*, **1**, 3–42.

Atherholt, T.B., Le Chevallier, M., Norton, W.D. and Rosen, J.S. (1998) Effect of rainfall on *Cryptosporidium* and *Giardia. Journal of the American Waterworks Association,* **90**, 66–80.

Barwick, R.S., Levy, D.A., Craun, G.F., Beach, M.J. and Calderon, R.L. (2000) Surveillance for waterborne disease outbreaks – United States, 1997–1998. *MMWR,* **49**(SS04), 1–35.

Bell, A., Guasparini, R., Meeds, D., Mathias, R.G. and Farley, J.D. (1993) A swimming pool associated outbreak of cryptosporidiosis in British Columbia. *Canadian Journal of Public Health*, **84**, 334–337.

Benenson, A.S. (1995) *Control of communicable diseases manual.* Sixteenth edition. Washington DC: American Public Health Association.

Bergquist, N.R., Stintzing, G., Smedman, L., Waller, T. and Andersson, T. (1984) Diagnosis of encephalitozoonosis in man by serological tests. *British Medical Journal*, **288**, 902.

Bing-Mu, H., Chihpin, H., Chih-Li, L.H., Yeong-Fua, H. and Yeh, J.H. (1999) Occurrence of *Giardia* and *Cryptosporidium* in the Kau-Ping river and its watershed in southern Taiwan. *Water Research,* **33**(11)**,** 2701–2707.

Bissessur, S. and Minderhoud, J.M. (1985) Two cases of schistosomiasis, *Clinical Neurology and Neurosurgery,* **87**(3), 213–217.

Cain, A.R.R., Wiley, P.F., Brownell, B. and Warhurst, D.C. (1981) Primary amoebic meningoencephalitis. *Archives of Disease in Childhood*, **56**, 140–143.

Castro-Hermida, J.A., González-Losada, Y.A., Mezo-Menéndez, M. and Ares-Mazás, E. (2002) A study of cryptosporidiosis in a cohort of neonatal calves. *Veterinary Parasitology,* **106**(1), 11–17.

Cerva, L. and Novak, K. (1968) Ameobic meningoencephalitis: sixteen fatalities. *Science,* **160**, 92.

Cetron, M.S., Chitsulo, L., Sullivan, J.J., Pilcher, J., Wilson, M., Noh, J., Tsang, V.C., Hightower, A.W. and Addiss, D.G. (1996) Schistosomiasis in Lake Malawi. *The Lancet,* **348**(9037), 1274–1278.

Chan, M.S., Medley, G.F., Jamison, D. and Bundy, D.A. (1994) The evaluation of potential global morbidity attributable to intestinal nematode infections. *Parasitology,* **109**, 373–387.

Checkley, W., Gilman, R.H., Epstein, L.D., Suarez, M., Diaz, J.F., Cabrera, L., Black, R.E. and Sterling, C.R. (1997) Asymptomatic and symptomatic cryptosporidiosis: Their acute effect on weight gain in Peruvian children. *American Journal of Epidemiology*, **45**, 156–163.

Chupp, G.L., Alroy, J., Adelman, L.S., Breen, J.C. and Skilnik, P.R. (1993) Mytositis due to Pleistophora (Microsporidia) in a patient with AIDS. *Clinical Infectious Diseases: An Official Publication of the Infectious Diseases Society of America,* **16**, 15–21.

Corachán, M., Almeda, J., Vinuesa, T., Valls, M.E., Mejias, T,. Jou, P., Biarnés, C., Pous, E., Vilana, R. and Gascón, J. (1997) Schistosomiasis imported by Spanish travelers: clinico-epidemiologic study of 80 cases. *Medica Clinica*, **108**(19), 721–725.

Cotte, L., Rabodonirina, M., Chapuis, F., Bailly, F., Bissule, F., Raynal., C., Gelas, P., Persat, F., Piens, M. and Trepo, C. (1999) Waterborne outbreak of intestinal microsporidiosis in persons with and without Human Immunodeficiency Virus infection. *The Journal of Infectious Diseases*, **180**, 2003–2008.

Craun, G.F., Hubbs, S.A., Frost, F., Calderon, R.L. and Via, S.H. (1998) Waterborne outbreaks of cryptosporidiosis. *Journal of the American Waterworks Association,* **90,** 81–91.

Cron, R.Q. and Sherry, D.D. (1995) Reiter's syndrome associated with cryptosporidial gastroenteritis. *Journal of Rheumatology,* **22,** 1962–1963.

Current, W.C. and Garcia, L.S. (1991) Cryptosporidiosis. *Clinical Microbiology Review,* **4,** 325–358.

De Jonckheere, J. (1971) Occurrence of *Naegleria* and *Acanthameoba* in aquaria. *Applied Environmental Microbiology,* **38**(1971), 590–593.

De Jonckheere, J. (1987) Epidemiology. In: *Amphizoic amoebae, human pathology.* (ed. E.G. Rondanelli) Piccin Nuova Libraria, Padova. pp. 127–147.

DeNapoli, T.S., Rutman, J.Y., Robinson, J.R. and Rhodes, M.M. (1996) Primary amoebic meningoencephalitis after swimming in the Rio Grande. *Texas Medicine,* **92**(10), 59–63.

Dillingham, R.A., Lima, A.A. and Guerrant, R.L. (2002) Cryptosporidiosis: Epidemiology and impact. *Microbes and Infection,* **4**(10), 1059–1066.

Dowd, S.E. (2002) *Microsporidia*: Occurrence, fate and methodologies. In: *Encyclopaedia of Environmental Microbiology,* Volume 4, (ed. Bitton, G.), John Wiley & Sons Inc., New York, USA.

Dowd, S.E., Gerba, C.P. and Pepper, I.L. (1998) Confirmation of the human-pathogenic Microsporidia *Enterocytozoon bieneusi, Encephalitozoon intestinalis* and *Vittaforma cornea* in water. *Applied and Environmental Microbiology,* **64**(9), 3332–3335.

Duma, R.J., Shumaker, J.B. and Callicott, J.H. (1971) Primary amoebic meningoencephalitis: A survey in Virginia. *Archives of Environmental Health,* **23,** 43–47.

Farthing, M.J.G. (1994) Giardiasis as a disease. In *Giardia: From molecules to disease.* (ed. R.C.A. Thompson, J.A. Reynoldson and A.J. Lymbery), pp. 15–37, Wallingford, CAB International, UK.

Fayer, R., Morgan, U. and Upton, S.J. (2000) Epidemiology of *Cryptosporidium*: transmission, detection, and identification. *International Journal of Parasitology.* **30,** 1305–1322.

Feldmeier, H., Poggensee, G., Krantz, I. and Helling-Giese, G. (1995) Female genital schistosomiasis. New challenges from a gender perspective. *Acta Tropica (Suppl.),* **47,** 2–15.

Ferreira, F.M.B., Bezerra, L., Bela, M., Santos, G., Bernardes, R.M.A., Avelino, I. and Sampaio Silva, M.L. (2001) Intestinal microsporidiosis: A current infection in HIV-seropositive patients in Portugal. *Microbes and Infection,* **3**(12), 1015–1019.

Ferreira, M.S. and Borges, A.S. (2002) Some aspects of protozoan infections in immunocompromised patients – a review. *Memorias do Instituto Oswaldo Cruz, Rio de Janeiro,* **97**(4), 443–457.

Field, A.S., Marriott, D.J., Milliken, S.T., Brew, B.J., Canning, E.U., Kench, J.G., Darveniza, P. and Harkness, J.L. (1996) Myositis associated with a newly described microsporidian, *Trachipleistophora hominis,* in a patient with AIDS. *Journal of Clinical Microbiology,* **34,** 2803–2811.

Flannagan, P.A. (1992) *Giardia* – diagnosis, clinical course and epidemiology – a review. *Epidemiology and Infection,* **109,** 1–22.

Fournier, S., Dubrou, S., Ligoury, O., Gaussin, F., Santillana-Hayat, M., Sarfati, C., Molina, JM. and Derouin, F. (2002) Detection of *Microsporidia, Cryptosporidia* and *Giardia* in swimming pools: a one-year prospective study. *FEMS Immunology and Medical Microbiology*, **33**, 209–213.

Fournier, S., Ligoury, O., Santillana-Hayat, M., Guillot, E., Sarfati, C., Dumoutier, N., Molina, J.M. and Derouin, F. (2000) Detection of *Microsporidia*, in surface water: A one-year follow-up study. *FEMS Immunology and Medical Microbiology*, **29**, 95–100.

Fowler, M. and Carter, R.F. (1965) Acute pyogenic meningitis probably due to *Acanthamoeba* sp.: A preliminary report. *British Medical Journal*, **5464**, 740–742.

Franzen, C. and Muller, A. (1999) *Cryptosporidia* and *Microsporidia* – waterborne diseases in the immunocompromised host. *Diagnostic Microbiology and Infectious Disease*, **34**, 245–262.

Franzen, C. and Muller, A. (2001) Microsporidiosis: Human diseases and diagnosis. *Microbes and Infection*, **3**(5), 389–400.

Furness, B.W., Beach, M.J. and Roberts, J.M. (2000) Giardiasis surveillance – United States, 1992–1997. *MMWR*, **49**(SS07), 1–13.

Gallaher, M.M., Herndon, J.L., Nims, L.J., Sterling, C.R., Grabowski, D.J. and Hull, H.F. (1989) Cryptosporidiosis and surface water. *American Journal of Public Health*, **79**, 39–42.

Gogate, A. and Deodhar, L. (1985) Isolation and identification of pathogenic *Naegleria fowleri* (aerobia) from a swimming pool in Bombay. *Transactions of the Royal Society of Tropical Medicine and Hygiene*, **79**(1), 134.

Gray, S.F., Gunnell, D.J. and Hatlen, J.B. (1994) Risk factors for giardiasis: a case-control study in Avon and Somerset. *Epidemiological Infection*, **113**, 95–102.

Gray, S.F. and Rouse, A.R. (1992) Giardiasis – a cause of traveller's diarrhoea. *Communicable Disease Report Review*, **2**(4), R45–R47.

Greensmith, C.T., Stanwick, R.S., Elliot, B.E. and Fast, M.V. (1988) Giardiasis associated with a water slide. *Pediatric Infectious Diseases*, **7**, 91–94.

Groseclose, S.L., Braithwaite, W.L., Hall, P.A., Knowles, C., Adams, D.A., Connor, F., Hester, M., Sharp, P., Anderson, W.J. and Fagan, R.F. (2002) Summary of notifiable diseases – United States 2000. *MMWR*, **49**(53), 1–102.

Guerrant, R.L., Kosek, M., Lima, A.A.M., Lorntz, B. and Guyatt, H.L. (2002) Updating the DALYs for diarrhoeal disease. *Trends in Parasitology*, **18**(5), 191–193.

Guerrant, D.I., Moore, S.R., Lima, A.A., Patrick, P.D., Schorling, J.B and Guerrant, R.L. (1999) Association of early childhood diarrhoea and cryptosporidiosis with impaired physical fitness and cognitive function four – seven years later in a poor urban community in north-east Brazil. *American Journal of Tropical Medicine and Hygiene*, **61**, 707–713.

Harter, L., Frost, F., Grunenfelder, G., Perkinis-Jones, K. and Libby, J. (1984) Giardiasis in an infant and toddler swim class. *American Journal of Public Health*, **74**, 155–156.

Hay, E.M., Winfield, J. and McKendrick, M.W. (1987) Reactive arthritis associated with *Cryptosporidium enteritis*. *British Medical Journal*, **295**, 248.

Health Canada (2001). Material data safety sheet – infectious substances. Available on-line. http://www.hc-sc.gc.ca/pphb-dgspsp/msds-ftss/index.html#menu.

Hill, J.S., Gaston, M. and Lillicrap, S. (2003) Arthritis associated with enteric infections. *Best Practice and Research Clinical Rheumatology*, **17**(2), 219–239.

Ho, B.S.W. and Tam, T.Y. (1998) Occurrences of *Giardia* cysts in beach water. *Water, Science and Technology*, **38**(12), 73–76.

Hoxie, N.J., Davis, J.P., Vergeront, J.M., Nashold, R.D. and Blair, K.A. (1997) Cryptosporidiosis-associated mortality following a massive waterborne outbreak in Milwaukee, Wisconsin. *American Journal of Public Health,* **87**(12), 2032–2035.

Huang, D.B., Chappell, C. and Okhuysen, M.D. (2004) Cryptosporidiosis in children. *Seminars in Pediatric Infectious Diseases,* **15**(4), 253–259.

Huffman, D.E., Gennaccaro, A., Rose, J.B. and Dussert, B.W. (2002) Low- and medium-pressure UV inactivation of microsporidia *Enterocytozoon intestinalis. Water Research,* **36**, 3161–3164.

Hunter P.R. (1998) *Waterborne Disease: Epidemiology and Ecology.* John Wiley & Sons, Chichester, UK.

Hutin, Y.J., Sombardier, M.N., Liquory, O., Sarfatei, C., Derouin, F. and Modai, J. (1998) Risk factors for intestinal microsporidiosis in patients with human immunodeficiency virus infection: a case-control study. *The Journal of Infectious Diseases,* **178**(3), 904–907.

IARC Working Group on the Evaluation of Carcinogenic Risks to Humans (1994) Evaluation of carcinogenic risks to humans: schistosomes, liver flukes and *Helicobacter pylori. IARC Monograph,* **61**, 26.

Islam, A. (1990) Giardiasis in developing countries. In: *Human parasitic diseases,* vol. 3, (ed. E.A. Meyer), pp. 235–266, Elsevier, Amsterdam, The Netherlands.

James, S. (1997) Emerging parasitic infections. *FEMS Immunology and Medical Microbiology,* **18**, 313–317.

Jariya, P., Makeo, S., Jaroonvesama, N., Kunaratanapruk, S., Lawhanuwat, C and Pongchaikul, P. (1983) Primary ameobic meningoencephalitis: a first reported case in Thailand. *Southeast Asian Journal of Tropical Medicine and Public Health,* **14**(4), 525–527.

Jeans, A.K. and Schwellnus, M.P. (1994) The risk of schistosomiasis in Zimbabwean triathletes. *South African Medical Journal,* **84**, 756–758.

Joce, R.E., Bruce, J., Kiely, D., Noah, N.D., Dempster, W.B., Stalker, R., Gumsley, P., Chapman, P.A., Norman, P., Watkins, J., Smith, H.V., Price, T.J. and Watts, D. (1991) An outbreak of cryptosporidiosis associated with a swimming pool. *Epidemiology and Infection,* **107**, 497–508.

John, D.T. (1982) Primary ameobic meningoencephalitis and the biology of *Naegleria fowleri. Annual Review of Microbiology,* **36**, 101–103.

Johnson, D.C., Reynolds, K.A., Gerba, C.P., Pepper, I.L. and Rose, J.B. (1995) Detection of *Giardia* and *Cryptosporidium* in marine waters. *Water Science and Technology,* **31**(5–6), 439–442.

Kadlec, V., Cerva, L. and Skvarova, J. (1978) Virulent *Naegleria fowleri* in an indoor swimming pool. *Science,* **201**, 1025.

Kilvington, S. and Beeching, J. (1995) Identification and epidemiological typing of *Naegleria fowleri* with DNA probes. *Applied and Environmental Microbiology,* **61**, 2071–2078.

Kloos, H., Higashi, G.I., Cattabni, J.A., Schlinski, V.D., Mansour, N.S. and Murrell, K.D. (1983). Water contact behaviour and schistosomiasis in an upper Egyptian village. *Social Science and Medicine,* **17**(9), 545–562.

Kosek, M., Alcantara, C., Lima, A. and Guerrant, R.L. (2001) Cryptosporidiosis: an update. *The Lancet Infectious Diseases,* **1**, 262–269.

Koudela, B., Kucerova, S. and Hudovic, T. (1999) Effect of low and high temperatures on infectivity of *Enterocytozoon cuniculi* spores suspended in water. *Folia Parasitologica,* **46**(3), 171–174.

Kramer, M.H., Herwaldt, B.L., Calderon, R.L. and Juranek, D.V.M. (1996) Surveillance for waterborne-disease outbreaks – United States, 1993–1994. *MMWR*, **45**(SS01), 1–33.

Kramer, M.H., Sorhage, F.E., Goldstein, S.T., Dalley, E., Wahlquist, S.P. and Herwaldt, B.L. (1998) First reported outbreak of cryptosporidiosis associated with a recreational lake. *Clinical Infectious Diseases: An Official Publication of the Infectious Diseases Society of America*, **26**(1), 27–33.

Lane, S. and Lloyd, D. (2002) Current trends in research into the waterborne parasite *Giardia*. *Critical Reviews in Microbiology*, **28**(2), 123–147.

Lares-Villa, F., de Jonckheere, J.F., de Moura, H., Rechi-Iruretoagoyena, A., Ferreira-Guerrero, E., Fernandez-Quintantilla, G., Ruiz-Matus, C. and Visvesvara, G.S. (1993) Five cases of primary amoebic meningoencephalitis in Mexicali, Mexico: A study of the isolates. *Journal of Clinical Microbiology*, **31**, 685–688.

Lawande, R., Macfarlane, J.T., Weir, W.R. and Awunor-Renner, C. (1979) A case of primary amebic meningoencephalitis in a Nigerian farmer. *The American Journal of Tropical Medicine and Hygiene*, **29**(1), 21–25.

Le Chevallier, M.W., Norton, W.D. and Lee, R.G. (1991) *Giardia* and *Cryptosporidium* spp. in filtered drinking water supplies. *Applied Environmental Microbiology*, **57**, 2617–2621.

Ledford, D.K., Overman, M.D., Gonzalvo, A., Cali, A., Mester, S.W. and Lockey, R.F. (1985) *Microsporidiosis myositis* in a patient with the acquired immunodeficiency syndrome. *Annals of Internal Medicine*, **102**, 628–630.

Lee, S.H., Levy, D.A., Craun, G.F., Beach, M.J. and Calderon, R.L. (2002) Surveillance for waterborne-disease outbreaks – United States, 1999–2000. *MMWR*, **51**(SS08), 1–28.

Levy, D.A., Bens, M.S., Craun, G.F., Calderon, R.L., Herwaldt, B.L. (1998) Surveillance for waterborne disease outbreaks – United States, 1995–1996. *MMWR*, **47**(SS–5), 1–34.

Lipp, E., Farrah, S.A. and Rose, J.B. (2001) Assessment and impact of microbial faecal pollution and human enteric pathogens in a coastal community. *Marine Pollution Bulletin*, **42**(4), 286–293.

Lorntz, B., Soares, A.M., Silva, R.P., Moore, S., Gansneder, B., Bovbjerg, V.E., Guyatt, H., Lima, A.M and Guerrant, R.L. (2000) Diarrhoea in first two years of life (ECD) is associated with increased age for grade (AFG) and age at starting school (AASS) 5–9 years later. *49th Annual Meeting of American Society of Tropical Medicine and Hygiene*, Houston, TX, USA.

MacKenzie, W.R., Kazmierczak, J.J. and Davis, J.P. (1995) An outbreak of cryptosporidiosis associated with a resort swimming pool. *Epidemiology and Infection*, **115**, 545–553.

Mandell, G.L., Douglas, R.G. and Bennett, J.E. (1995) *Principles and Practice of Infectious Diseases*, 4th edn, Churchill Livingstone, New York.

Martinez, A.J. (1993) Free-living amoebas: infection of the central nervous system. *Mt Sinai Journal of Medicine*, **60**, 271–278.

Martinez, A.J. and Janitschke, K. (1985) *Acanthamoeba*, an opportunistic microorganism: a review. *Infection*, **13**(6), 251–257.

Martinez, A.J. and Visvesvara, G.S. (1991) Laboratory diagnosis of pathogenic free-living ameobas: *Naegleria*, *Acanthamoeba*, and *Leptomyxid*. *Clinics in Laboratory Medicine*, **11**, 861–872.

Martinez, A.J. and Visvesvara, G.S. (1997) Free-living, amphizoic and opportunistic amoebas. *Brain Pathology*, **7**(1), 583–598.

Matsubayashi, H., Koike, T., Mikata, T. and Hagiwara, S. (1959) A case of Encephalitozoon-like body infection in man. *Archives of Pathology*, **67**, 181–187.

McAnulty, J.M., Fleming, D.W. and Gonzalez, A.H. (1994) A community-wide outbreak of cryptosporidiosis associated with swimming at a wave pool. *Journal of the American Medical Association,* **272**, 1597–1600.

McGarvey, S.T., Zhou, X.N., Willingham, A.L., Feng, Z. and Olveda, R. (1999) The epidemiology and host-parasite relationships of *Schistosoma japonicum* in definitive hosts. *Parasitology Today,* **15**(6), 214–215.

McKerrow, J.H. and Salter, J. (2002) Invasion of skin by *Schistosoma* cercariae. *Trends in Parasitology,* **18**(5), 193–195.

Morales Gomez, M.A. (2004) Highly active antiretroviral therapy and cryptosporidiosis. *Parassitologia,* **46**(1–2), 95–99.

Mota, P., Rauch, C.A. and Edberg, S.C. (2000) *Microsporidia* and *Cyclospora*: epidemiology and assessment of risk from the environment. *Critical Reviews in Microbiology* **26**(2), 69–90.

Nath, G., Choudhury, A.M., Shukla, B.N., Singh, T.B. and Reddy, D.C. (1999) Significance of *Cryptosporidium* in acute diarrhoea in north-eastern India. *Journal of Medical Microbiology,* **48**(6), 523–526.

Ndamba, J., Makaza, N., Munjoma, M., Gomo, E. and Kaondera, K.C. (1993) The physical fitness and work performance of agricultural workers infected with *Schistosoma mansoni* in Zimbabwe. *Annals of Tropical Medicine and Parasitology,* **87**, 553–561.

Ndyomugyenyi, R. and Minjas, J.N. (2001) Urinary schistosomiasis in schoolchildren in Dar-es-Salaam, Tanzania, and the factors influencing its transmission. *Annals of Tropical Medicine and Parasitology,* **95**(7), 697–706.

Neal, K.R., and Slack, R.C.B. (1997) Risk factors for *Giardia* infection – more than just drinking the water. Recreational use of water in the United Kingdom and abroad is a route of infection. *Proceedings of the Society for Social Medicine Conference, York, UK.* Society for Social Medicine.

O'Donoghue, P.J. (1995) *Cryptosporidium* and cryptosporidiosis in man and animals. *International Journal of Parasitology,* **25**, 139–195.

Ofoezie, I.E., Christensen, N.O. and Madsen, H. (1998) Water contact patterns and behavioural knowledge of schistosomiasis in south west Nigeria. *Journal Biosocial Science,* **30**, 254–259.

Pernin, P. and Riany, A. (1978) Study on the presence of 'free-living amoebae in the swimming-pools of Lyon. *Annales de Parasitologie Humaine et Comparee,* **53**(4), 333–344.

Poggensee, G. and Feldmeier, H. (2001) Female genital schistosomiasis: facts and hypotheses. *Acta Tropica,* **79**, 193–210.

Porter, J.D., Ragazzoni, H.P., Buchanon, J.D., Wakin, H.A., Juranek, D.D. and Parkin, W.E. (1988) *Giardia* transmission in a swimming pool. *American Journal of Public Health,* **78**, 659–662.

Puech, M.C., McAnulty, J.M., Lesjak, M., Shaw, N., Heron, L. and Watson, J.M. (2001) A state-wide outbreak of cryptosporidiosis in New South Wales associated with swimming at public pools. *Epidemiology and Infection,* **126**(3), 389–396.

Quinn, R.W. (1971) The epidemiology of intestinal parasites of importance in the United States. *Southern Medical Bulletin,* **59**, 29–30.

Radke, M.G., Ritchie, L.S. and Rowan, W.B. (1961) Effects of water velocities on worm burdens of animals exposed to *Schistosoma mansoni* cercariae under laboratory and field conditions. *Experimental Parasitology,* **11**, 323–331.

Rivera, F., Cerva, L., Martinez, J., Keleti, G., Lares, F., Ramirez, E., Bonilla, P., Graner, S.R., Saha, A.K. and Glew, R.H. (1990) *Naegleria lovaniensis tarasca* new subspecies, and the *purepecha* strain, a morphological variant of *N. loveaniensis*, isolated from natural thermal waters in Mexico. *Journal of Protozoology*, **37**, 301–310.

Rivera, F., Ramirez, E., Bonilla, P. (1993) Pathogenic and free-living amoebae isolated from swimming pools ad physiotherapy tubs in Mexico. *Environmental Research,* **62**, 43–52.

Rivera, F., Ramirez, P., Vilaclara, G., Robles, E. and Medina, F. (1983) A survey of pathogenic and free-living amoebae inhabiting swimming pool water in Mexico City. *Environmental Research,* **32**(1), 205–211.

Rodriguez, R., Mendez, O., Molina, O., Luzardo, G., Martinez, A.J., Visvesvara, G.S and Cardozo J. (1998) Central nervous system infection by free-living amoebas: report of 3 Venezuelan cases. *Revista de Neurologia,* **26**(154), 1005–1008.

Rose, J.B., Huffman, D.E. and Gennaccaro, A. (2002) Risk and control of waterborne cryptosporidiosis**.** *FEMS Microbiology Reviews*, **26**(2), 113–123.

Sadaka, H.A., el-Nassery, S.F., abou Samra, L.M. and Awadalla, H.N. (1994) Isolation and identification of free-living amoebae from some water sources in Alexandria. *Journal of the Egyptian Society of Parasitology*, **24**(2), 247–257.

Savioli, L., Renganathan, E., Montresor, A., Davis, A. and Behbehani, K. (1997) Control of schistosomiasis—a global picture. *Parasitology Today* **13**(11), 444–448.

Shepherd, R.C., Smail, P.J. and Sinha, G.P. (1989) Reactive arthritis complicating cryptosporidial infection. *Archives of Disease in Childhood,* **64**, 743–744.

Sing, A., Bechtold, S., Heesemann, J., Belohradsky, B.H. and Schmidt, H. (2003) Reactive arthritis associated with prolonged cryptosporidial infection. *Journal of Infection*, **47**(2), 181–184.

Sirinavin, S., Jariya, P., Lertlaituan, P., Chuahirun, S. and Pongkripetch, M. (1989) Primary amoebic meningoencephalitis in Thailand: report of a case and review literatures. *Journal of the Medical Association of Thailand,* **72**(1), 174–176.

Slifko, T.R., Smith, H.W. and Rose, J.B. (2000) Emerging parasite zoonoses associated with water and food. *International Journal for Parasitology*, **30,** 1379–1393.

Smith, H.V. and Rose, J.B. (1990) Waterborne cryptosporidiosis. *Parasitology Today*, **6,** 8–12.

Stuart, J.M., Orr, H.J., Warburton, F.G., Jeyakanth, S., Pugh, C., Morris, I., Sarangi, J. and Nichols, G. (2003) Risk factors for sporadic giardiasis: A case-control study in South-western England. *Emerging Infectious Diseases,* **9**(2), 229–233.

Taylor, M.B., Becker, P.J., Van Rensburg, E.J., Harris, B.N., Bailey, I.W. and Grabow, WOK. (1995) A serosurvey of water-borne pathogens amongst canoeists in South Africa. *Epidemiology and Infection,* **115,** 299–307.

Terada, S., Reddy, K.R., Jeffers, L.J., Cali, A. and Schiff, E.R. (1987) Microsporidian hepatitis in the acquired immunodeficiency syndrome. *Annals of Internal Medicine,* **107,** 61–62.

Thompson, R.C.A., Hopkins, R.M. and Homan, W.L. (2000) Nomenclature and genetic groupings of *Giardia* infecting mammals. *Parasitology Today,* **16**, 210–213.

Tzipori, S. and Ward, H. (2002) Cryptosporidiosis: Biology, pathogenesis and disease. *Microbes and Infection*, **4**(10), 1047–1058.

Upatham E.S. (1976) Field studies on the bionomics of the free-living stages of St Lucian *Schistosoma mansoni*. *International Journal of Parasitology,* **6**, 239–245.

Useh, M.F. and Ejezie, G.C. (1999) School-based schistosomiasis control programmes: a comparative study on the prevalence and intensity of urinary schistosomiasis among

Nigerian school-age children in and out of school. *Transactions of the Royal Society of Tropical Medicine and Hygiene,* **93**(4), 387–391.

Vakil, N.B., Schwartz, S.M., Buggy, B.P., Brummitt, C.F., Kherellah, M., Letzer, D.M., Gilson, I.H. and Jones, P.G. (1996) Biliary cryptosporidiosis in HIV-infected people after the waterborne outbreak of cryptosporidiosis in Milwaukee. *New England Journal of Medicine,* **334**, 19–23.

Valenzuela, G., Lopez-Corella, E. and De Jonckheere, J.F. (1984) Primary amoebic meningoencephalitis in a young male from north-western Mexico. *Transactions of the Royal Society of Tropical Medicine and Hygiene,* **78**(4), 558–559.

Van der Werf, M.J., de Vlas, S. Brooker, S.J., Looman, C.W., Nagelkerke, N.J., Habbema, J.D. and Engels, D. (2003) Quantification of clinical morbidity associated with schistosome infection in sub-Saharan Africa. *Acta Tropica,* **86**(2–3), 125–139.

Watson, D., Asmuth, D. and Wanke, C. (1996) Environmental risk factors for acquisition of microsporidiosis in HIV-infected patients. *Clinical Infectious Diseases: An Official Publication of the Infectious Diseases Society of America,* **23**, 903.

Weiss, L.M. (2001) Microsporidia: emerging pathogenic protists. *Acta Tropica,* **78**, 89–102.

Wellings, F.M., Amuso, P.T., Chang, S.L. and Lewis, A.L. (1977) Isolation and identification of pathogenic *Naegleria* from Florida lakes. *Applied Environmental Microbiology,* **34**, 661–667.

WHO (2004a) *Guidelines for drinking-water quality.* 3rd edition. Volume 1, Recommendations. World Health Organization, Geneva.

WHO (2004b)
http://www.who.int/vaccine_research/documents/new_vaccines/en/index5.html.

WHO (2005) *Guidelines for safe recreational-water environments,* vol. 2 *Swimming pools, spas and similar recreational water environments.* WHO, Geneva.

Winchester, R., Bernstein, D.H., Fischer, H.D., Enlow, R. and Solomon, G. (1987) The co-occurrence of Reiter's syndrome and acquired immunodeficiency. *Annals of Internal Medicine,* **106**, 19–26.

Yachnis, A.T., Berg, J., Martinez-Salazar, A., Bender, B.S., Diaz, L., Rojiani, A.M., Eskin, T.A. and Orenstein, J.M. (1996) Disseminated microsporidiosis especially infecting the brain, heart and kidneys. Report of a newly recognised pansporoblastic species in two symptomatic AIDS patients. *American Journal of Clinical Pathology,* **106**, 535–543.

Yoder, J.S., Blackburn, B.G., Craun, G.F., Hill, M.P.H. and Levy, D.A. (2004) Surveillance for waterborne-disease outbreaks associated with recreational water – United States, 2000–2002. *MMWR Surveillance Summaries,* **53**(SS08), 1–22.

Zender, H.O., Arrigoni, E., Eckert, J. and Kapanci, Y. (1989) A case of *Encephalitozoon cuniculi* peritonitis in a patient with AIDS. *American Journal of Clinical Pathology,* **92**, 352–356.

Zu, S.X., Li, J.F., Barrett, L.J., Fayer, R., Shu, S.Y., McAuliffe, J.F., Roche, J.K. and Guerrant, R.L. (1994) Seroepidemiologic study of *Cryptosporidium* infection in children from rural communities of Anhui, China and Fortaleza, Brazil. *The American Journal of Tropical Medicine and Hygiene,* **51**(1), 1–10.

6

Viruses

This chapter summarises the evidence for viral illnesses acquired through ingestion or inhalation of water or contact with water during water-based recreation. The organisms that will be described are: adenovirus; coxsackievirus; echovirus; hepatitis A virus; and hepatitis E virus. The following information for each organism is presented: general description, health aspects, evidence for association with recreational waters and a conclusion summarising the weight of evidence.

HUMAN ADENOVIRUS

Credibility of association with recreational water: Strongly associated

I Organism

Pathogen

Human adenovirus

Taxonomy

Adenoviruses belong to the family Adenoviridae. There are four genera: *Mastadenovirus, Aviadenovirus, Atadenovirus* and *Siadenovirus.* At present 51 antigenic types of human adenoviruses have been described. Human adenoviruses have been classified into six groups (A–F) on the basis of their physical, chemical and biological properties (WHO 2004).

Reservoir

Humans. Adenoviruses are ubiquitous in the environment where contamination by human faeces or sewage has occurred.

Distribution

Adenoviruses have worldwide distribution.

Characteristics

An important feature of the adenovirus is that it has a DNA rather than an RNA genome. Portions of this viral DNA persist in host cells after viral replication has stopped as either a circular extra chromosome or by integration into the host DNA (Hogg 2000). This persistence may be important in the pathogenesis of the known sequelae of adenoviral infection that include Swyer-James syndrome, permanent airways obstruction, bronchiectasis, bronchiolitis obliterans, and steroid-resistant asthma (Becroft 1971; Tan *et al.* 2003). They are unusually resistant to chemical or physical agents and adverse pH conditions, allowing for prolonged survival outside of the body. Adenovirus has been shown to be resistant to both tertiary treatment and UV radiation of urban wastewater (Thompson *et al.* 2003; Thurston-Enriquez *et al.* 2003).

II Health aspects

Primary disease symptoms and sequelae

Adenoviruses are frequent causes of fevers, upper respiratory tract symptoms and conjunctivitis and produce infections that are usually mild and self limiting.

Adenoviral lower respiratory tract infections are infrequent, sporadic and most commonly associated with adenovirus types 3, 5 and 7 (Mandell 2000; Murtagh *et al.* 1993). Epidemic keratoconjunctivitis is associated with adenovirus serotypes 8, 19, and 37. Acute respiratory disease is most often associated with adenovirus types 4 and 7. Enteric adenoviruses 40 and 41 cause gastroenteritis, usually in children (Wilhelmi *et al.* 2003). Of the human adenoviruses belonging to the B subgenera, it is known that adenovirus types 3, 7, and 11 cause conjunctivitis (Kitamura 2001). Adenovirus type 3 and 7, which belong to the B1 group, cause inflammation of the upper respiratory tract and pneumonia in addition to conjunctivitis (Murtagh and Kajon 1997), while adenovirus type 11, which belongs to Group B2, causes diseases such as cystitis and nephritis (Kitamura 2001). It has been suggested that there is a possible connection between adenovirus type 36 and obesity (Powledge *et al.* 2004).

For some adenovirus serotypes, the clinical spectrum of disease associated with infection varies depending on the site of infection; for example, infection with adenovirus 7 acquired by inhalation is associated with severe lower respiratory tract disease, whereas oral transmission of the virus typically causes no or mild disease.

Many of the adenovirus serotypes can multiply in the small intestine, but only types 40 and 41 have been strongly associated with gastroenteritis (Grimwood *et al.* 1995). Adenovirus is considered to be second only to rotavirus in terms of its significance as a cause of childhood gastroenteritis (Crabtree *et al.* 1997). Studies covering the analysis of about 5000 faecal specimens during the period 1981–1996 indicate that adenoviruses contributed 3% to 9% of the gastroenteritis cases admitted to Australian hospitals. The majority of the cases were associated with young children and involved serotype 41 (40% to 80%) and to a lesser extent, serotype 40 (less than 20%). Seasonal patterns of the virus genotypes were evident, with type 41 being prevalent in late autumn and type 40 remaining prevalent year-round (Grimwood *et al.* 1995; Palambo and Bishop 1996).

Infection with adenovirus is usually acquired during childhood. Acute lower respiratory tract infections in children is a major worldwide health problem (Murray and Lopez 1996). In Argentina, viral infections have been shown to contribute to between 20% and 30% of all cases of acute lower respiratory tract infections in children and in a community setting, approximately 14% of cases have been shown to be attributable to adenovirus (Avila *et al.* 1989; Videla *et al.* 1998). This is higher than that reported in other countries. In Sweden for example, adenoviruses are reported to be responsible for 5% of acute lower respiratory infections in children under 4 years of age who require hospitalisation (Sharp and Wadell 1995).

Although most adenovirus infections are mild, adenovirus is included in this review because rarely, these infections may be fatal and there are a number of sequelae associated with the viral infection. Acute necrotizing bronchitis and bronchiolitis may develop in children and in debilitated and immunocompromised patients (Edwards *et al.* 1985; Ruuskanen *et al.* 1985; Zahradnik *et al.* 1980). These infections may result in complications including recurrent wheezing, bronchiectasis and obliterative bronchiolitis (Simila *et al.* 1981; Sly *et al.* 1984; Hardy *et al.* 1988; Macek *et al.* 1994; Arce *et al.* 2000). Furthermore, adenoviral infections in lung transplant recipients may produce a rapidly progressive course leading to premature death (Ohori *et al.* 1995; Simsir *et al.* 1998). Unlike other viral pneumonitides (e.g. herpes simplex virus, cytomegalovirus), no specific treatment for adenovirus pneumonitis exists.

Viquesnel *et al.* (1997) report a case of severe adenovirus type 7 pleuropneumonia in an immunocompetent adult. The treatment required a mechanical ventilation with tracheostomy. The sequela was a restrictive respiratory insufficiency. Zarraga *et al.* (1992) report a case of adenovirus type 3 infection in a previously healthy adult woman that resulted in severe pulmonary complications.

There are many cases of adenovirus-related illness in military recruits documented in the literature, some of these resulted in deaths. Two fatal cases of adenovirus-related illness in previously health military recruits in the state of Illinois, United States in 2000 were reported (Anonymous 2001). Both recruits died. The first case developed viral encephalitis, bronchiolitis obliterans and organizing pneumonia. The second case developed acute respiratory distress syndrome. Although the serotype responsible was not identified, serotype 7 has been most commonly associated with meningitis and encephalitis (Yamadera *et al.* 1998). It is thought that adenovirus may have been a co-morbidity factor in these cases.

Exposure/mechanism of infection

Exposure and infection are likely to be via several routes. The most common method of transmission is via the faecal–oral route, with food and water as possible vectors (Mickan and Kok 1994). In addition the virus may be spread through contaminated surfaces, such as sharing of towels at swimming pools, or sharing of goggles. Airborne spread through coughing and sneezing is also common. Outbreaks of adenovirus-associated respiratory disease have been more common in the late winter, spring, and early summer; however, adenovirus infections can occur throughout the year.

Disease incidence

The exact prevalence and incidence of adenoviral infections are unknown, because most cases are seen by general practitioners and optometrists. Adenovirus is a very common infection, estimated to be responsible for between 2% and 5% of all respiratory infections. In winter, infection with type 4 or 7 causes recognisable illness in military recruits, with about 25% requiring hospitalisation for fever and lower respiratory tract disease (Berkow *et al.* 2004).

Crabtree *et al.* (1997) calculated annual risks of infection from adenovirus in recreational water to be as high as 1/1000 for a single exposure.

Incubation period

Incubation periods are generally less than ten days (Foy 1997; Gaydos 1999) but may be up to 24 days (Hunter 1998).

Infectivity

An infective dose of less that 150 plaque forming units has been reported when given intra-nasally (Health Canada 2002).

Sensitive groups

All ages are susceptible to adenovirus infections. Infections in the newborn may be serious, from meningitis and myocarditis to generalised systemic infection including hepatic dysfunction, even death (Cherry 1990; Abzug and Levin 1991). There are a few case reports of serious pneumonia caused by adenovirus in the newborn (Bhat *et al.* 1984; Sun and Duara 1985).

Young children are particularly sensitive to adenovirus types 1,2,3, and 5 which are the most common cause of tonsillopharyngitis. Adenovirus infections have a greater severity of illness in the immunocompromised (e.g. AIDS patients and transplant recipients; Crabtree *et al.* 1997; Madhi *et al.* 2000). Hierholzer (1992) report a case-fatality rate of 53% for adenovirus infection in people with reduced immune function due to cancer treatment.

III Evidence for association of adenovirus with recreational waters

In seawater, the enteric adenoviruses have been shown to be substantially more stable than either polio 1 or HAV. They are reported to be more resistant to inactivation by UV than enteroviruses and sometimes are detected at higher levels in polluted waters (Crabtree *et al.* 1997). This suggests that the enteric adenoviruses may survive for prolonged periods in water, representing a potential route of transmission (Enriquez and Gerba 1995).

Epidemics of pharyngoconjunctival fever are associated with waterborne transmission of some adenovirus types. These are generally recorded from inadequately chlorinated swimming pools (Heinz *et al.* 1977) and small lakes. Most surveillance studies of adenovirus infections have been conducted in developed countries.

Foy *et al.* (1968) reported an outbreak of pharyngoconjunctival fever in two childrens' swimming teams after exposure to unchlorinated water. The attack rates in the two teams were 65% and 67% respectively. Although the virus could not be isolated from the pool water, the author speculated that faecal contamination of the unchlorinated water could have been the source of the contamination.

In 1974, Caldwell *et al.* reported an outbreak of conjunctivitis associated with adenovirus type 7 in seven members of a community swimming team in Kansas, United States. Viral culture of conjunctival and throat swabs of eight cases were positive for adenovirus type 7. In this case the pools' chlorinator and filter had failed.

Adenovirus type 4 was the causative agent of an outbreak of pharyngoconjunctivitis in users of a private swimming pool in Georgia, United States in the summer of 1977. Among members the attack rate was significantly higher in those who had used the pool (P<0.001). The virus was detected in samples of pool water and isolated from 20 of 26 swab specimens. It was found that there were inadequate levels of chlorine in the pool water (D'Angelo *et al.* 1979).

Martone *et al.* (1980) report a second outbreak in the same year and locality linked to adenovirus type 3 and swimming pool use. At least 54 cases were identified with symptoms such as sore throat, fever, headache and anorexia. Conjunctivitis affected 35% of the individuals. The outbreak coincided with a temporary defect in the pool filter system and inadequate maintenance of the chlorine levels.

Turner *et al.* (1987) report an outbreak of adenovirus type 7a infection associated with a swimming pool in which it was subsequently discovered the chlorinator had temporarily malfunctioned. Symptoms of pharyngitis were reported in 77 individuals. A telephone survey indicated that persons who swum at the community swimming pool were more likely to be ill than those that did not. Those who swallowed water were more likely to be ill than those that did not (relative risk 2.1; P<0.01).

An outbreak of pharyngoconjunctival fever at a summer camp in North Carolina, United States was reported in July 1991 (Anonymous 1992). An epidemiological investigation identified the cause as pharyngoconjunctival fever associated with infection with adenovirus type 3. Approximately 700 persons swam every day in a one-acre man-made pond into which well water was continuously pumped. The attack rate for campers who swam daily (48%) did not differ significantly from that for campers who swam less than once per week (65%; relative risk 0.8). The attack rate for staff who swam was higher than that for staff who did not swim (77% versus 54%; relative risk 1.4). Of the 221 campers and staff members interviewed, 75 reported they had shared a towel with another person. Towel sharing increased the risk for illness (11 of 12 who shared versus 31 of 63 who did not; relative risk 1.9%). Of viral cultures obtained from 25 ill persons, 19 grew adenovirus serotype 3. A concentrated sample of pond water drawn approximately six feet below the surface yielded adenovirus serotype 3.

An outbreak of pharyngoconjunctivitis amongst competitive swimmers in southern Greece caused by adenovirus is reported by Papapetropoulou and Vantarakis (1998). At least 80 persons showed symptoms of fever, sore throat, conjunctivitis, headache and abdominal pain. It was shown the outbreak was due to adenovirus in a poorly chlorinated pool.

Harley *et al.* (2001) report an outbreak of pharyngoconjunctival fever in a primary school in North Queensland, Australia. There was a strong correlation between the development of symptoms and having been swimming on a recent school camp. At the peak of the outbreak 40% of students were absent from the school. Although adenovirus could not be isolated from the swimming pool water from the camp, it was found that the swimming pool was not adequately chlorinated or maintained and it was concluded that it was probable that adenovirus infection was transmitted via the swimming pool water.

IV Conclusions

There are 51 types of adenovirus and the diseases resulting from infections include conjunctivitis, pharyngitis, pneumonia, acute and chronic appendicitis, bronchiolitis, acute respiratory disease, and gastroenteritis. Adenovirus infections are generally mild; however, there are a number of fatal cases of infection reported in the literature. Transmission of adenovirus in recreational waters, primarily inadequately chlorinated swimming pools, has been documented via faecally-contaminated water and through droplets, although no fatal cases attributable to recreational waters have been documented in the literature.

Human adenovirus	Epidemiological evidence linking recreational water use with illness	Evidence from outbreak data of illness associated with recreational water	Documented cases of illness associated with recreational water	Documented cases of sequelae (in any situation)
	√	√	√	√

COXSACKIEVIRUS

Credibility of association with recreational water: Probably associated

I Organism

Pathogen

Coxsackievirus A and B

Taxonomy

The coxsackieviruses belong to the Picornaviradae family. They are divided into two groups, A and B. There are 23 serotypes of coxsackie A viruses and at least six serotypes of coxsackie B virus (King *et al.* 2000). Those from the group B are associated with more severe illness.

Reservoir

Human, spread by direct contact with nasal and throat secretions from an infected person, faecal–oral route, inhalation of infected aerosols.

Distribution

Coxsackievirus has worldwide distribution, with increased frequency occurring in warm months in temperate climates.

Characteristics

The picornaviruses are small RNA-containing viruses, 25–30 nm in diameter. They can remain viable for many years at extremely low temperatures (between minus 20 $^{\circ}$C and 70 $^{\circ}$C, and for weeks at 4 $^{\circ}$C, but lose infectivity as the temperature rises.

II Health aspects

Primary disease symptoms and sequelae

The clinical manifestations of coxsackievirus infections range from inapparent infection in most persons (76%; Minor 1998) to uncommon and fatal disease. Coxsackieviruses are the most common cause of non-polio enterovirus infections (Mena *et al.* 2003).

Mild illnesses include common cold and rashes, hand, foot and mouth disease and herpangina. Children between one and seven years of age have the highest incidence of herpangina. Most cases occur in the summer months, either sporadically or in outbreaks. The illness is characterised by an abrupt fever together with a sore throat, dysphagia, excessive salivation, anorexia, and malaise. About 25% of patients suffer from vomiting and abdominal pain. Vesicles appear on the anterior tonsillar pillars. Headache and myalgia are common in some outbreaks. The fever lasts between one and four days, local and systemic symptoms begin to improve in four to five days, and total recovery is usually within a week. In rare cases aseptic meningitis, and parotitis may develop (Hlavová 1989).

Coxsackievirus A10 has been associated with lymphonodular pharyngitis (Hunter 1998). This is generally seen in children but may also affect young adults. Symptoms include fever, mild headache, myalgia, and anorexia due to a sore throat. The symptoms generally last between 4 and 14 days. Complications are not common.

Hand, foot and mouth disease is associated predominately with coxsackieviruses A16 and A5 and occurs most frequently in children (Tsao *et al.* 2002). The disease is associated with low-grade fever at the onset. Sore throat or sore mouth are the usual presenting symptoms. Skin lesions typically occur, although they are not always present. The entire illness lasts between four and eight days. Although hand, foot and mouth disease is generally mild, associated features include aseptic meningitis, paralytic disease, and fatal myocarditis.

Coxsackievirus A24 has been identified as the causal agent for acute haemorrhagic conjunctivitis (Yin-Murphy and Lim 1972).

Since the 1960s, it has been suggested that group B coxsackieviruses are the most frequent viral etiological agent associated with heart diseases including myocarditis, pericarditis and endocarditis (Burch and Giles 1972; Koontz and Ray 1971; Pongpanich *et al.* 1983; Ward 2001; Gauntt and Huber 2003), causing more than 50% of all cases of viral myocarditis (Ali and Abdel-Dayem 2003). The presence of heart-specific autoantibodies in the sera of some patients with coxsackievirus B3-induced myocarditis has suggested that autoimmunity is a sequela of viral myocarditis (Wolfgram *et al.* 1985). Potentially, autoimmunity can develop in genetically predisposed individuals whenever damage is done to the cardiac tissue.

Sporadic cases of paralysis have been associated with coxsackievirus infections. The serotypes that are most often implicated are coxsackieviruses B2-6 (Kono *et al.* 1977). The disease is milder than poliomyelitis and paralysis is usually not permanent.

Coxsackievirus has been implicated in cases of arthritis and arthralgias (Franklin 1978; Lucht *et al.* 1984). Gullain-Barré syndrome has been reported in a small number of patients associated with coxsackievirus serotypes A2, A5 and A9 (Dery *et al.* 1974).

Coxsackieviruses can, albeit rarely, cause encephalitis (McAbee and Kadakia 2001). Around 70% of all meningitis cases are attributed to enteroviruses, in particular coxsackievirus types A7, A9 and B2-5 (Mena *et al.*1999).

Many epidemiologic investigations have supported the involvement of coxsackievirus B in the etiology of pancreatitis and insulin dependent diabetes mellitus (IDDM) (Ramsingh *et al.* 1997; Jaekel *et al.* 2002; Horwitz *et al.* 2004). It has been suggested the virus can precipitate the symptoms of IDDM in individuals who already have advanced beta-cell damage (Hyöty *et al.* 2003). Molecular analyses revealed positive associations between the presence of enteroviral mRNA and the development of beta cell autoimmunity (Andréoletti *et al.* 1998), and type 1 diabetes (Clements *et al.* 1995; Hou *et al.* 1994).

The majority of IDDM cases manifest before the age of 30 years and the incidence is highest in childhood and puberty (Leslie and Elliot 1994). Around 50% of children with IDDM have antibodies to coxsackievirus and it has been documented that enteroviruses and especially coxsackie B, have been implicated in between 20 and 34% of all human pancreatitis cases (Mena *et al.* 2000).

In utero infection of the placenta with coxsackievirus is associated with the development of severe respiratory failure and central nervous system sequelae in the newborn (Euscher 2001).

There are a few reports suggesting an association of coxsackievirus with rheumatic fever (Suresh *et al.* 1989; Zaher *et al.* 1993; Górska *et al.* 1998).

Aronson and Phillips (1975) suggest that an association exists between coxsackievirus B5 infections and acute oliguric renal failure.

Exposure/mechanisms of infection

Coxsackievirus infections can be spread directly from person-to-person via the faecal–oral route or contact with pharyngeal secretions (Hunter 1998). In addition the virus may be spread by aerosols or through water. The virus infects the mucosal tissues of the pharynx, gut or both and enters the bloodstream where it gains access to target organs such as the meninges, myocardium and skin.

Disease incidence

The exact incidence and prevalence of coxsackievirus infections are not known but they are extremely common. Data on the seroprevalence of coxsackie B2, B3, B4 and B5 virus in the Montreal area of Canada were obtained during an epidemiological study on water-related illnesses (Payment 1991). These are shown in Table 6.1.

Table 6.1 Seroprevalence (expressed as a percentage) to coxsackieviruses in a French-Canadian population (Adapted from Payment 1991)

Serogroup	Age groups (years)				
	9–19	20–39	40–49	50–59	60+
B2	51	60	67	66	60
B3	51	64	63	55	60
B4	44	80	77	74	80
B5	58	74	61	62	20

Other than paralytic polio, diseases associated with enterovirus infections, are not normally notifiable. In the United States the National Enterovirus Surveillance System collects information on enterovirus serotypes and monitors temporal and geographic trends. Each year in the United States, an estimated 30 million nonpoliomyelitis enterovirus infections cause aseptic meningitis, hand, foot and mouth disease; and non specific upper respiratory disease. During 2000 and 2001, coxsackievirus B5 accounted for 11.9% of reports with an identified serotype, and coxsackievirus B5 accounted for 6.3% (Anonymous 2002). The findings were consistent with previous observations – coxsackievirus A9, B2 and B4 have appeared consistently among the 15 most common serotypes each year between 1993 and 1999 (Anonymous 1997; 2000).

Incubation period

The incubation periods vary. For coxsackievirus type A9, between 2 and 12 days; for types A21 and B5, between three and five days (Hoeprich 1977).

Infectivity

The infectious dose is likely to be low – less than 18 infectious units by inhalation (Coxsackie A21; Health Canada 2001).

Sensitive groups

Children and the immunocompromised are most sensitive to coxsackievirus infections (Mandell 2000).

III Evidence for association of coxsackievirus with recreational waters

There have been two documented recreational water outbreaks associated with coxsackievirus. Transmission of coxsackieviruses from lake waters has been documented for coxsackievirus B5 (Hawley *et al.* 1973) and coxsackie A16 (Denis *et al.* 1974).

Hawley *et al.* (1973) described an outbreak of coxsackievirus B5 infection at a summer camp in northern Vermont, United States in 1972. The virus was isolated from 13 individuals, one boy was admitted to hospital with conjunctivitis, sinusitis and meningitis. There is no epidemiological evidence to prove that swimming was associated with the transmission of the illness. Coxsackievirus was isolated from the lake.

Epidemiological studies linking a suspected viral outbreak with water are difficult because limited waterborne viral outbreaks usually occur at distance from the original source of contamination (WHO 1979). However, D'Alessio *et al.* (1981) studied 296 children with symptoms typical of an enteroviral infection, and 679 controls with no symptoms. Viruses were isolated from 287 cases, group A coxsackieviruses were isolated from 45 of these and group B coxsackievirus from 29. A history of swimming was obtained from all cases and controls. It was concluded that children from whom an enterovirus was isolated were more likely to have swum at a beach than controls. Those who only swum in a swimming pool were not at increased risk. Case children from whom no virus was isolated did not differ from healthy controls.

In May 1992, a 20-year old man developed nausea following a surfing outing in Malibu. His symptoms grew progressively worse and coxsackie B virus was isolated from him. He subsequently died from damage to his heart, caused by the virus. Although it was not proved that the virus was contracted whilst surfing, it was thought that this was the case (Dorfman 2004).

IV Conclusions

Although there have been very few outbreaks of coxsackievirus linked to recreational water recorded, and epidemiological evidence remains scarce the virus has been frequently isolated from marine and freshwaters. As with other viruses (HAV, adenovirus and echovirus) transmission of the virus is possible and biologically plausible in susceptible persons.

Coxsackievirus	Epidemiological evidence linking recreational water use with illness	Evidence from outbreak data of illness associated with recreational water	Documented cases of illness associated with recreational water	Documented cases of sequelae (in any situation)
	√	√	√	√

ECHOVIRUS

Credibility of association with recreational water: Probably associated

I Organism

Pathogen

The enterovirus – Echovirus.

Taxonomy

The echoviruses belong to the family Picornaviridae, genus *Human Enterovirus B*. Recently the classification of the Picornaviridae has been updated and there are now a total of 28 distinct echovirus sero-types known to infect humans (King *et al.* 2000).

Reservoir

Humans. Echoviruses are excreted in the faeces of infected individuals. Among the types of viruses detectable by conventional cell culture isolation, enteroviruses, including echoviruses are generally the most numerous in sewage, water resources and treated drinking-water supplies (WHO 2004).

Distribution

Echovirus is distributed worldwide.

Characteristics

The echoviruses are small, linear, positive sense RNA-containing viruses. The viruses have an icosahedral structure with a diameter of 27 nm.

II Health aspects

Primary disease symptoms and sequelae

Non-polio enteroviruses, which include all coxsackieviruses and echoviruses, are predominantly organisms of the gastrointestinal tract with transmission by the faecal–oral route. In addition, transmission can take place via the respiratory route.

Initially it was believed that echoviruses primarily caused acute aseptic meningitis syndromes, pleurodynia, exanthems, pericarditis, non-specific febrile illness and occasional fulminant encephalomyocarditis of the newborn. It is now apparent that their spectrum of disease is much broader; there may be long-term sequelae and some infections may trigger chronic active disease processes. Diaz-Horta *et al.* (2001); Hyöty and Taylor (2002) and Cabrera-Rode (2003) amongst others have shown that echovirus infection might be capable of inducing a process of autoimmune beta-cell damage supporting the hypothesis that enterovirus infections are important risk factors for the development of Type 1 diabetes. Enteroviral infections during pregnancy have been implicated as a risk factor for the later development of IDDM (Otonkoski *et al.* 2000).

Several studies have shown that echovirus 7 may cause sporadic cases or small outbreaks of severe or fatal encephalitis in otherwise healthy children. Echovirus 7 was reported by Madhaven and Sharma (1969) as the predominant virus isolated from 26 clinically diagnosed cases of encephalitis in Pondicherry, India. Several of these cases died within a few hours of admission but no further clinical details were available. Fatal echovirus 7 infection has been reported in infants during outbreaks in special care nurseries (Kazi *et al.* 1988; Wreghitt *et al.* 1989; See Lum *et al.* 2002).

Echovirus 9 and echovirus 30 have been frequently associated with outbreaks of aseptic meningitis (Andersson *et al.* 1975; Anonymous 1995; Uysal *et al.* 2000), with the milder central nervous system disease being attributed to echovirus 7. Echovirus 7-associated brain stem encephalomyelitis has been well documented in Bulgaria (Chumakov *et al.* 1979), Malaysia, Taiwan and Western Australia (See Lum *et al.* 2002).

Ho-Yen *et al.* (1989) describe a maculopapular rash in a nine-month-old boy who succumbed to hepatic failure due to echovirus infection.

Published reports and international data from WHO support the suggestion that echovirus types 6 and 19 share the potentiality of type-B coxsackieviruses for causing acute carditis and pleurodynia (Bell and Grist 1974).

An association between echovirus type 33 infection and acute flaccid paralysis has recently been reported by Grimwood *et al.* (2003).

Exposure/mechanism of infection

Some viral replication occurs in the nasopharynx after ingestion, with spread to regional lymph nodes. However, most innoculum is swallowed and reaches the lower gastrointestinal tract, where the virus binds to specific receptors on enterocytes. The virus crosses the intestinal epithelium, and reaches the Peyer patches in the lamina propria mucosae where the virus undergoes substantial multiplication. Many secondary infection sites, including the central nervous system, liver, spleen, bone marrow, heart, and lungs occur. Additional replication at these sites causes a major viremia that coincides with onset of clinical disease, usually four to six days after exposure. The delayed appearance of central nervous system disease symptoms suggests viral spread can occur during both the minor and the major viremia.

Infections involving a single serotype may vary widely in their presentation; multiple serotypes can produce the same clinical syndrome.

Disease incidence

Echovirus and other enteroviruses account for 30 million infections in the United States each year (WHO 2004). It has been suggested that the high prevalence of echovirus 13 (responsible for aseptic meningitis), considered previously a rare serotype, indicates it is an emerging epidemic type (Inge *et al.* 2003). Many echovirus infections are asymptomatic (approximately 43%; Minor 1998), therefore it is difficult to determine the true incidence of infection. Echovirus is a common cause of summer respiratory infections in children, they occur with a higher prevalence in summer and autumn months (Mandell 2000).

Incubation period

The incubation period for echovirus is difficult to establish because both symptomatic and healthy individuals spread the virus. Incubation is believed to range between two days and two weeks (Mandell 2000).

Infectivity

The infectious dose is estimated to be in the region of 10^5 to 10^6 infectious particles (Hunter 1998).

Sensitive groups

Disease depends on the age, gender and immune status of the host, as well as the subgroup and serotype of the infecting strain.

Although echovirus infections can occur in all age groups, incidence inversely relates to age; specific antibodies directly increase with time. Several studies performed during epidemics and for surveillance show that infants become infected at significantly higher rates than older children and adults. The incidence of some syndromes, such as myo- or pericarditis, is greatest in neonates (Minor 1998). Some forms of echovirus disease such as meningitis and neonatal sepsis have been reported to be far more common among male patients (Froeschle *et al.* 1966).

III Evidence for association of echovirus with recreational waters

A number of studies have isolated echovirus from freshwater recreational waters, swimming pools and waste waters (Marzouk *et al.* 1980; Keswick *et al.* 1981; Rose *et al.* 1987). Application of polymerase chain reaction technology has indicated the presence of echovirus in seawater samples (Muscillo *et al.* 1995).

In 1992, an outbreak of gastroenteritis in a village in Northern Ireland was reported (Kee *et al.* 1994). Forty-six people reported symptoms of vomiting, diarrhoea and headache soon after swimming in an outdoor swimming pool. It was discovered that 34 swimmers had become ill and one swimmer had vomited in the pool. Other cases were reported after the swimming incident. Individuals who had swallowed water were more likely to become ill than those who had not. Echovirus 30 was isolated from the case that had vomited and from six other cases. Although chlorine levels had been maintained at the correct levels, they were inadequate to control the risk of infection from the pool.

IV Conclusions

As with the other enteroviruses (coxsackievirus and adenovirus) discussed in this review, there are few published cases of infection by echovirus in recreational water, those that are recorded are primarily from swimming pool water. The most likely source of the virus is through faecal contamination, although secretions from the eyes or throat are possible.

There are likely to be many unreported cases of infection with echovirus since outbreaks of acute gastrointestinal infections with unknown etiology are common, with the symptomatology of the illness frequently being suggestive of viral, including echoviral, infections.

Echovirus	Epidemiological evidence linking recreational water use with illness	Evidence from outbreak data of illness associated with recreational water	Documented cases of illness associated with recreational water	Documented cases of sequelae (in any situation)
	√	√	√	√

HEPATITIS A

> Credibility of association with recreational waters: Probably associated

I Organism

Pathogen

Hepatitis A virus

Taxonomy

HAV is a small, single-stranded RNA virus belonging to the family Picornaviridae. It is the only member of the *Hepatovirus* genus.

Reservoir

Humans are the only known reservoir. The occurrence of the virus in raw water sources reflects epidemiological features such as the outbreak in a particular community.

Distribution

Worldwide. HAV is most common in tropical and subtropical countries. Table 6.2 shows the levels of endemicity in different regions of the world.

Table 6.2 Worldwide endemicity of HAV infection (WHO 2003)

HAV endemicity	Regions by epidemiological pattern	Average age of patients (years)	Most likely mode of transmission
Very high	Africa, parts of south America, the Eastern Mediterranean and South-East Asia regions	under 5	Person-to-person Contaminated food and water
High	Amazon Basin (Brazil), China and Latin America	5–14	Person-to-person Outbreaks/contaminated food or water
Intermediate	Southern and eastern Europe, some regions of the Eastern Mediterranean region	5–24	Person-to-person Outbreaks/contaminated food or water
Low	Australia, United States, western Europe	5–40	Common source outbreaks
Very low	Northern Europe and Japan	over 20	Exposure during travel to endemic areas, uncommon source

Characteristics

The virus particle is spherical, 27–28 nm in diameter and lacks an envelope. The virus is stable at pH 3, resistant to intestinal enzymes and a temperature of 60 °C for 10 hours (Percival *et al.* 2004). The virus remains stable for months after storage at room temperature and in water, sewage and shellfish (Sobsey *et al.* 1998).

II Health aspects

Primary disease symptoms and sequelae

HAV infection causes a prodromal illness of fever, nausea, loss of appetite, abdominal pain and mild gastrointestinal upset, followed by jaundice. In young children the disease is often asymptomatic (Cuthbert 2001) and the severity of disease increases with age. Hollinger and Ticehurst (1996) predict the mortality rate for patients of 40 years to be 2.1% whereas for patients of 14 years it is 0.1%. Only around 25% of patients become jaundiced and this develops between two and seven days after the development of the prodromal illness. The first signs of jaundice are a darkening of the urine and a lightening of stools. The patient may also show signs of a yellowing of the eyes and an enlarging of the liver. The patient probably remains infectious for seven days after the start of the jaundice (Hunter 1998). The majority of adults who become infected are symptomatic, with acute cholestatic jaundice (Ledner *et al.* 1985). Relapsing hepatitis is also seen in between 6% and 10% of cases (Schiff 1992; Ciocca 2000).

Fulminant hepatitis is the most severe form of infection. The case-fatality rate is 80% (Hoofnagle *et al.* 1995), but fulminant hepatitis is rare (less than 1% of cases overall), although rates are higher with increasing age and where patients have liver disease. Although children appear to be at a lower risk of symptomatic infection and of severe liver disease than adults, they occasionally develop liver failure leading to the requirement for a liver transplant. Children are also at risk from death. The average age at the onset of fulminant hepatic failure in children is reported to be six and a half years (Debray *et al.* 1997). Immunity after infection protects against re-infection and appears to be retained for life.

Hepatic insufficiency is the most severe complication of HAV. It is more commonly observed in adult patients. In most cases, the outcome of hepatic insufficiency is rapidly favourable. In rare cases, hepatic insufficiency progresses and encephalopathy subsequently occurs. At this stage, emergency liver transplantation may be necessary. Apart from hepatic insufficiency, complications include cholestasis (impairment of bile flow resulting in accumulation in the blood of substances normally secreted in bile such as bilirubin, bile salts and cholesterol), which may last for several months, and relapsing disease. Cholestatic HAV is characterised by persistent jaundice associated with pruritus, anorexia and weight loss. Recovery usually occurs after several weeks or months without treatment. Relapsing HAV is characterised by rising levels of serum enzyme, persistence of IgM anti-HAV, and possibly recurrent faecal virus shedding.

Extrahepatic manifestations of HAV include temporary skin rash and arthralgias. Documented cases of arthritis and cutaneous vasculitis associated with cryoglobinaemia are rare and HAV has never been documented to evolve into chronic hepatitis (Schiff 1992). One case of adult Still's disease triggered by vaccination to HAV and Hepatitis B is reported in the literature by Grasland *et al.* (1998).

Exposure/mechanism of infection

HAV is very infectious and spread in a variety of ways – through the person-to-person or environmental routes. Direct person-to-person transmission through the faecal–oral route is probably the most common route of transmission; however outbreaks associated with raw or undercooked shellfish, harvested from polluted waters, sexual-contact and blood transfusions have also been described (Hunter 1998).

Since humans are considered to be the only natural host for HAV (Hunter 1998), waterborne transmission of viral hepatitis must be preceded by human faecal contamination. The virus passes through the stomach, where it replicates in the lower intestine, and then passes to the liver where replication is more rapid. The virus is excreted from the liver in the bile and contaminates the faeces.

Due to the nature of the ecology of HAV any surface water that is subject to faecal or sewage contamination will be at risk of contamination by HAV, depending on the prevalence of the disease in the population polluting the water body. HAV is excreted in large numbers in faeces of infected persons (symptomatic and asymptomatic), (at least 10^8 particles or 10^6 infectious virons/g), and the virus remains infectious for a long time since it is highly resistant to environmental conditions (Debord and Buisson 1998).

HAV seems to follow minor cyclic patterns, with peaks occurring during the autumn and winter, possibly as a result of exposure during the summer in endemic areas. In the United States, for example, nationwide outbreaks occur approximately every ten years (WHO 2000).

Disease incidence

Worldwide, there are at least 1.5 million cases of HAV annually (WHO 2002), although this is likely to be an underestimate. HAV imposes a large economic burden throughout the world – on average, adults suffering from HAV miss 30 days of work. It has been estimated that medical treatment and work loss account for an estimated $500 million annually in the United States (Berge *et al.* 2000) between $1.5 and $3 billion annually worldwide (André 1995; Hollinger and Ticehurst 1996).

In developed countries where HAV infection is no longer primarily in childhood and sanitation and hygienic conditions are good, infection rates of HAV are low, although disease may occur among specific risk groups such as travellers. In 1990, 7545 cases were reported to the PHLS from England and Wales with 260 deaths between 1989 and 1999 recorded attributable to HAV (Crowcroft *et al.* 2001).

Incubation period

The mean incubation period for HAV is 28 days (range 15–50 days; Crowcroft *et al.* 2001). Peak infectivity occurs two weeks before the onset of jaundice and falls quickly after that. Children and infants may excrete HAV for longer than adults.

Infectivity

HAV is not readily detectable by routine cell culture procedures and therefore the epidemiology of the virus as well as its incidence and behaviour in the environment are not well known. It is known that it is highly infectious – one outbreak caused by the consumption of infected clams resulted in 300,000 cases in 1988 in Shanghai, China – and it is thought that the minimal infectious dose is extremely low, possibly as low as a single infectious particle (Zhi-Yi *et al.* 1992).

Sensitive groups

Risks for acquiring HAV are widespread in developing countries and it is a significant cause of death and socio-economic loss in many parts of the world, especially where there are poor levels of sanitation. Reported disease rates in these areas are low and outbreaks are rare since infection is usually acquired in childhood as an asymptomatic or mild infection (WHO 2000).

III Evidence for association of hepatitis A with recreational waters

The potential risk of transmission of HAV by the waterborne route has been known for over 20 years. A number of studies have isolated HAV from surface waters which could be used for recreational purposes (Cecuk *et al.* 1993; Bryan *et al.* 1974; Chapman 1976; Rosenberg *et al.* 1980; Ramia 1985; Panà *et al.* 1987; Shuval 1988; Taylor *et al.* 2001) and therefore may pose a potential health risk. Several studies have reported HAV in the effluent of treatment plants implying a potential risk posed by the discharge of viruses. Hugues *et al.* (1988) found HAV in three samples of effluent in southern France; Panà *et al.* (1987) isolated HAV from polluted river water in Italy; Schvoerer *et al.* (2000) report three strains of HAV isolated from sewage treatment plants and neighbouring rivers in south-western France although none were isolated from the designated bathing areas nearby.

Surveillance data

HAV is a notifiable disease in many countries. The total number of cases of HAV is thus readily available from a number of countries. However, it is not easy to associate cases with recreational use of water and no data from the surveillance centres contacted for the purposes of this research confirmed a link.

Published cases of hepatitis A associated with recreational waters

There are a few published cases of HAV associated with water used for recreational purposes (Table 6.3).

Table 6.3 Published cases of hepatitis A associated with water used for recreational purposes.

Date of outbreak/case	Country	Reference	Notes
1969	United States	Bryan et al. 1974	14 cases of HAV in boy scouts camping in a lake recreation area.
1976	United States	Chapman 1976	26 individuals affected after playing in a polluted stream running through a housing development.
1992	United States	Mahoney et al. 1992	20 people aged between 4 and 36 years contracted HAV after using a swimming pool.
1994	France	Garin et al. 1994	Exposure to enteroviruses and HAV among divers in environmental waters in France.
1995	South Africa	Taylor et al. 1995	Implicates faecally polluted water as a possible source of HAV in South African canoeists.
1997	Australia	Tallis and Gregory 1997	An outbreak of HAV associated with a hot tub.

Bryan et al. (1974) report 14 cases of HAV in a group of boy scouts who attended a camp in South Carolina, United States in August 1969. The camp was based on an island in a recreational lake. An epidemiological investigation was carried out and it was concluded that the common-source outbreak of HAV was limited to individuals who had attended the camp and that exposure to the source of infection occurred on the island. Samples of lake water obtained at both the recreation area and at the campsite showed gross contamination with coliform organisms. Water from a protected well was transported to the camp and stored for drinking but water was also taken from the lake to douse the fire and many scouts admitted to being unaware of the difference in the water and may have drunk the water from the lake. Scouts also recalled swallowing quantities of lake water while swimming. Seven of the eight individuals who drank or accidentally swallowed large quantities of lake water became ill, whereas only two of the ten people not drinking the water contracted HAV. It was not possible to demonstrate the presence of HAV in the lake water nor was it possible to find the source(s) which could have contaminated the lake.

Chapman (1976) reports a series of epidemics of HAV in a community in Salishan, Washington, United States, between 1958 and 1974. The patients were primarily young children or young adults. The source of the infection was traced to a creek into which sewage effluent which could not be absorbed by the soil during extended rainfall was released. Children from the area were known to play in the ravine and the creek thereby exposing themselves to sewage effluent and HAV.

In 1989 it was reported that three children from two families in Louisiana, United States, had HAV. They had no common exposures except to a commercial campground which included two heated pools, a non-heated tub, and a wading pool, as well as a pool which was only open to members. Mahoney *et al.* (1992) carried out an epidemiological study to identify the cause of the outbreak. Among 822 campers during one weekend, 20 developed HAV. A strong association was found between illness and exposure to two of the public pools. At the time of the outbreak the weather was hot and many people were swimming which may have depleted the free chlorine in the pools, although this was not proven. It is suggested that contamination could have occurred via a mixture of raw sewage with pool water during routine pool maintenance. The management at the pools reported that faecal contamination of the pools by swimmers was not uncommon.

Garin *et al.* (1994) conducted an epidemiological study of HAV and enteroviruses in a military diving training school between September 1991, and August 1992, at the Rhone and Saône rivers (20 km north of Lyon, France), Lake Bourget (100 km east of Lyon) and swimming pools of the diving school. Water samples were taken from each of the sites during training sessions and analysed for enterovirus, HAV and faecal bacteria. Blood samples were taken from the divers on the day of arrival in the school, at the end of the training course and one month after departure. Although enteroviruses were isolated no HAV or seroconversion to HAV was observed.

Research by Gammie and Wyn-Jones (1997) revealed a statistical correlation between surfing and exposure to HAV. The study investigated both surfers and windsurfers and compared their immune status to HAV. A higher rate of immunity was found in surfers and the study showed that the risk of surfers acquiring HAV was three times greater than windsurfers. HAV immunity was correlated with the total number of exposures in the surfing population. The authors recommended that surfers be offered vaccination to ensure they are protected from the risk of contracting HAV.

Anecdotal cases/other sources

Surfers Against Sewage, a pressure group based in the United Kingdom, have compiled a database of cases of illnesses reportedly acquired whilst using United Kingdom waters for recreational purposes. In all cases the patient saw a doctor. Ninety per cent of the reported cases resulted in a hospital visit. Ten cases of HAV were reported to Surfers Against Sewage between 1989 and 1996 (Table 6.4).

Table 6.4 Cases of self-reported hepatitis A acquired in waters used for recreational purposes, United Kingdom, and reported to Surfers Against Sewage, 1995–1996.

Location	Year	Activity being reported as resulting in contraction of HAV
Bude, Devon	1989	Swimming
Holywell Bay, Cornwall	1994	Surfing
Littlehampton, West Sussex	1995	Swimming
Eastbourne, East Sussex	1995	Windsurfing
Gwithian, Cornwall	1995	Surf-skiing
Broadhaven, Wales	1995	Not specified
Broadhaven, Wales	1996	Not specified
Pendennis, Cornwall	1996	Not specified
Gwenver, Cornwall	1996	Not specified
Hurley Wier, River Thames	1996	Kayaking

IV Conclusions

HAV has been isolated from surface waters which may be used for recreational purposes and a number of cases of HAV have been documented associated with recreational water users.

Fulminant hepatitis is rare and has not been reported in any cases linked with the use of recreational waters. No cases of sequelae of HAV contracted through the use of recreational waters were found in the literature and the probability of developing long-term sequelae is low. The acute disease is usually moderately severe and of moderate duration but risk of death is low.

Hepatitis A	Epidemiological evidence linking recreational water use with illness	Evidence from outbreak data of illness associated with recreational water	Documented cases of illness associated with recreational water	Documented cases of sequelae (in any situation)
	√	√	√	√

HEPATITIS E

Credibility of association with recreational waters: Probably associated

I Organism

Pathogen

Hepatitis E virus

Taxonomy

Although it is related to the alpha-virus superfamily, the HEV is classified as a separate hepatitis-E-like viruses genus (Worm *et al.* 2002).

Reservoir

HEV is acquired directly from infected persons by the faecal–oral route or by close contact, or by consumption of contaminated food or drinking-water. Zoonotic transmission has been suggested (Tei *et al.* 2003).

Distribution

HEV is most common where sanitary conditions are poor and the safety of drinking-water is not well controlled. HEV was first identified in India in 1955, and has since been recognised in the Eastern Mediterranean Region, South Asian countries, in northern and western Africa, the Russian Federation, and in China. Outbreaks have been reported from Algeria, Bangladesh, Borneo, China, Côte d'Ivoire, Egypt, Ethiopia, Greece, India, Indonesia, the Islamic Republic of Iran, Jordan, Kazakstan, Libya, Mexico, Myanmar, Nepal, Nigeria, Pakistan, Somalia, eastern Sudan, Tajikistan, The Gambia, Thailand, Turkmenistan, Uzbekistan, and Vietnam (Bradley 1992; Harrison 1999). Epidemics are more common where the climate is hot and are rare in temperate climates.

Characteristics

HEV is a non-enveloped, polydenylated, single-stranded, positive-sense RNA virus (Hunter 1998).

II Health aspects

Primary disease symptoms and sequelae

HEV is an acute viral hepatitis with abrupt onset of fever, malaise, nausea and abdominal discomfort, followed by the development of jaundice a few days later. Infection in very young children is usually mild or asymptomatic; older children are at risk of symptomatic disease. The disease is more severe in young to middle aged adults (Harrison 1999), with illness lasting several weeks and recovery taking several months. Occasionally, a fulminant form of hepatitis develops; case-fatality is greater than 2% for those over 40 years of age and 4% for those over 60. The disease is usually mild in nature and is self-limiting, without any long-term sequelae except where fulminant hepatitis cases occur in pregnancy (Khuroo *et al.* 1981; Mirghani *et al.* 1992). In these cases mortality may reach 20% in the third trimester. High infant mortalities of up to 33% due to premature deliveries are recorded (Bradley 1992; Lemon 1995; Purcell 1995) although opinions differ over the maternal and foetal outcome of pregnancies associated with viral hepatitis (Jaiswal *et al.* 2001). Gerba *et al.* (1996) estimate that pregnant mothers suffer from a case-fatality ratio from HEV infections ten times greater than the general population during waterborne disease outbreaks.

Although sequelae are not common, acute pancreatitis has been reported as associated with HEV. Six cases were reported by Mishra *et al.* (1999). Common cholestatic jaundice can persist for several weeks.

Exposure/mechanisms of infection

HEV is predominantly transmitted via the enteric route (Metcalf *et al.* 1995). Studies have documented the presence of HEV in swine (Meng *et al.* 1997; Chandler 1999) and chicken (Haqshenas *et al.* 2001), and therefore contamination of sewage with animal-derived faeces may represent another important source of transmission of such viruses to humans and animals consuming contaminated water. This may have implications for recreational water management. Outbreaks associated with contaminated water or food supplies have also been described. There are no documented cases of person-to-person transmission (Karetnyi *et al.* 1999).

Most cases of acute HEV in the United States, central and western Europe have been reported amongst travellers returning from high HEV-endemic areas, although this is not always the case (Zuckerman 2003).

It is suspected that in some countries the cases of HEV infection could be causatively related to the consumption of shellfish cultivated in sewage-polluted waters (Balayan 1993).

Disease incidence

Little information was found regarding the disease incidence or prevalence. During the last two decades, the following number of cases were reported by WHO: 119,000 cases in China between 1986 and 1988, 11,000 cases in

Somalia, and about 4,000 cases in Mexico between 1988 and 1989, 79,000 cases in Kanpur, India, in 1991 (WHO 2002).

Incubation period

The incubation period for HEV ranges from three to eight weeks, with a mean of 40 days (Lemon 1995; Purcell 1995).

Infectivity

The infectious dose of HEV is unknown.

Sensitive groups

Young children and pregnant women are more susceptible to symptomatic HEV infections.

III Evidence for association of hepatitis E with recreational waters

Contaminated water is recognised as an important vehicle for the transmission of several viral and other diseases and the sewage is the largest biological sink. Viruses, such as HEV excreted in faeces and urine constitute significant proportion of pathogens present in the sewage (Kopecka *et al.* 1993). Contamination of recreational water with sewage therefore could lead to infections among those consuming such water in sufficient quantities. However, no reports of HEV linked to recreational water use were found in the published literature although there are many reports of HEV in persons who have drunk sewage-contaminated or inadequately treated water taken from rivers. Two cases of HEV described below are reported in persons who swam in the River Ganges but also drank unboiled and unfiltered water whilst in India. It is unclear which was the source of HEV.

During June 1991, a high school student, who had been born in India and had lived in the United States since the age of one year, travelled to Varanasi, India. Before his trip he received prophylactic immunoglobulin for HAV. Approximately four weeks after his arrival in India, he developed diarrhoea, sore throat, fever, and general malaise and subsequently had weight loss of 20 pounds. On return to the United States, one week after onset of his symptoms, physical examination revealed scleral icterus and a mildly tender and enlarged liver. Although serologic markers for hepatitis A, B, and C were negative, anti-HEV was detected (Anonymous 1993). The patient denied a history of alcohol abuse, intravenous drug use, blood transfusions, or known contact with anyone diagnosed with hepatitis virus. The patient reported that during his stay in Varanasi, most of the drinking water he consumed was boiled or commercially filtered. However, he reported he occasionally drank unboiled or unfiltered water, and he swam in the Ganges River. The patient recovered fully (Anonymous 1993).

From mid-June through the end of July 1989, a male college student travelled to Pakistan, Nepal, and India. Before his trip, he received prophylactic HAV immunoglobulin. After his return to the United States, he developed nausea, fever, epigastric discomfort, and marked fatigue. Physical examination revealed scleral icterus and a mildly tender and enlarged liver. Although tests for serologic markers for hepatitis A, B, and C were negative, anti-HEV was detected.

The patient denied a history of alcohol abuse, intravenous drug use, blood transfusions, or known contact with anyone diagnosed with hepatitis. The patient reported that during his trip abroad he did not boil his drinking water (he treated the water with iodine), and he swam in the Ganges River. The patient recovered fully (Anonymous 1993).

The only other case found relates to a case of HEV in a man in California, United States. Approximately one month before the onset of his illness, he had gone camping with his children in the Sierra Nevada mountains for one week. At the campsite they drank unboiled water from a well that was located approximately 60 feet from a toilet. The patient, but not his children, also drank water from a lake where he was fishing. His children did not develop any illness after the trip. The source cannot be established but was clearly within California. Although the patient had been exposed to well and lake water during the incubation period, other modes of transmission (e.g. contaminated food) were also possible (Reichier *et al.* 2000).

IV Conclusions

The hepatitis E virus has been isolated from surface waters which may be used for recreational purposes.

Fulminant hepatitis is rare. No cases of sequelae of HEV contracted through the use of recreational waters were found in the literature and the probability of developing long-term sequelae is low. The acute disease is usually moderately severe and of moderate duration but risk of death is low except where cases occur during pregnancy.

Hepatitis E	Epidemiological evidence linking recreational water use with illness	Evidence from outbreak data of illness associated with recreational water	Documented cases of illness associated with recreational water	Documented cases of sequelae (in any situation)
			Not definitive	√

REFERENCES

Abzug, M.J. and Levin, M.J. (1991) Neonatal adenovirus infection: Four patients and review of literature. *Pediatrics*, **87**, 890–897.

Ali, M.A. and Abdel-Dayem, T.M.K. (2003) Myocarditis: an expected health hazard associated with water resources contaminated with Coxsackie viruses type B. *International Journal of Environmental Health Research*, **13**(3), 261–270.

Andersson, S.O., Bjorksten, B. and Burman, L.A. (1975) A comparative study of meningoencephalitis epidemics caused by echovirus type 7 and coxsackievirus type B5. *Scandanavian Journal of Infectious Diseases*, **7**, 233–237.

André, F.E. (1995) Approaches to a vaccine against hepatitis A: development and manufacture of an inactivated vaccine. *Journal of Infectious Diseases*, **171**(Supplement 1), S33–S39.

Andréoletti, L., Hober, D., Hober-Vandenberghc, C., Isabelle Fajardy, I., Belaich, S., Lambert, V., Vantyghem, M-C., Lefebvre, J. and Wattre, P. (1998) Coxsackie B virus infection and beta cell autoantibodies in newly diagnosed IDDM adult patients. *Clinical and Diagnostic Virology*, **9**,125–133.

Anonymous (1992) Outbreak of phayrngoconjunctival fever at a summer camp – North Carolina, 1991. *MMWR*, **41**(19), 342–344.

Anonymous (1993) Hepatitis E among U.S. travelers, 1989–1992. *MMWR*, **42**(01), 1–4.

Anonymous (1995) Outbreak of aseptic meningitis – Whiteside County, Illinois. *MMWR*, **46**(10), 221–224.

Anonymous (1997) Nonpolio enterovirus surveillance – United States, 1993–1996. *MMWR*, **46**(32), 748–750.

Anonymous (2000) Enterovirus surveillance – United States 1997–1999. *MMWR*, **49**(40), 913–916.

Anonymous (2001) Two fatal cases of adenovirus-related illness in previously healthy young adults – Illinois, 2000. *MMWR*, **50**(26), 553–555.

Anonymous (2002) Enterovirus surveillance – United States, 2000–2001. *MMWR*, **51**(46), 1047–1049.

Arce, J.D.V., Mondaca, R.A., Mardones, R., Velozo, L.F. and Parra, G.O. (2000) Secuelas post-infection pro adenovirus en Ninos: evaluacion con tomografia computada. *Revista Chilena de Radiologia*, **8**(4), 154–163.

Aronson, M.D. and Phillips, C.A. (1975) Coxsackie B5 infections in acute oliguric renal failure. *The Journal of Infectious Diseases*, **132**(3), 303–306.

Avila, M.M., Carballal, G., Rovaletti, H. Ebekian, B., Cusminsky, M. and Weissenbacher, M. (1989) Viral etiology in acute lower respiratory infections in children from a closed community. *The American Review of Respiratory Disease,* **140**, 634–637.

Balayan, M.S. (1993) Hepatitis E virus infection in Europe: regional situation regarding laboratory diagnosis and epidemiology. *Clinical and Diagnostic Virology,* **1**(1), 1–9.

Becroft, D.M.O. (1971) Bronchiolitis obliterans, bronchiectasis, and other sequelae of adenovirus type 21 infection in young children. *Journal of Clinical Pathology*, **24**, 72–82.

Bell, E.J. and Grist, N.R. (1970) Echovirus, carditis and acute pleurodynia. *The Lancet,* **295**(7642), 326–328.

Berge, J.J., Drennan, D.P., Jacobs, R.J., Jakins, A., Meyerhoff, A.S. and Stubblefield, W. (2000) The cost of hepatitis A infections in American adolescents and adults in 1997. *Hepatology*, **31**, 469–473.

Berkow, R., Beers, M.H. and Burs, M.H. (2004) *Infectious Diseases.* In: *Merck Manual Diagnosis and Therapy.* Seventeenth Edition. Merck & Co. Inc. New Jersey, USA.

Bhat, A.M., Meny, R.G., Aranas, E.H. and Yehia, F. (1984) Fatal adenoviral (type 7) respiratory disease in neonates. *Clinical Pediatrics,* **23**, 409–411.

Bradley, D.W. (1992) Hepatitis E: epidemiology, aetiology and molecular biology. *Review of Medical Virology,* **2**, 18–28.

Bryan, J.A., Lehmann, J.D., Setiady, I.F. and Hatch, M.H. (1974) An outbreak of hepatitis A associated with recreational lake water. *American Journal of Epidemiology,* **99**(2), 145–154.

Burch, G.E. and Giles, T.D. (1972) The role of viruses in the production of heart disease. *American Journal of Cardiology*, **29**, 231–240.

Cabrera-Rode, E., Sarmiento, L., Tiberti, C., Molina, G., Barrios, J., Hernández, D., Díaz-Horta, O. and Di Mario, U. (2003) Type 1 diabetes islet associated antibodies in subjects infected by echovirus 16. *Diabetologia,* **46**(10), 1348–1353.

Caldwell, G.G., Lindsey, N.J., Wulff, H., Donnelly, D.D. and Bohl, F.N. (1974) Epidemic with adenovirus type 7 acute conjuctivitis in swimmers. *American Journal of Epidemiology,* **99**, 230–234.

Cecuk, D., Kruzic, V., Turkovic, B. and Grce, M. (1993) Human viruses in the coastal environment of a Croatian harbour. *Revue d'Epidemiologie et de Santé Publique*, **41**(6), 487–493.

Chandler, J.D., Riddell, M.A. Li, F. Love, R.J. and Anderson, D.A. (1999) Serological evidence for swine hepatitis E virus infection in Australian pig herds. *Veterinary Microbiology,* **68**(1–2), 95–105.

Chapman, L. (1976) Hepatitis attributed to a polluted stream. *Journal of Environmental Health,* **38**(4), 238–241.

Cherry, J.D. (1990) Enteroviruses. In: *Infectious disease of the fetus and newborn infant* (ed. J.S. Remington, and J.O. Klein), pp. 325–366, Saunders, Philadelphia, USA.

Chumakov, M., Voroshilova, M., Shindarov, L., Lavrova, L., Gracheva, I., Koroleva, G., Vasilenko, S., Brodvarova, I., Nikolova, M., Gyurova, S., Gacheva, M., Mitov, G., Ninov, N., Tsylka, E., Robinson, I., Frolova, M., Bashkirtsev, V., Martiyanova, L. and Rodin, V. (1979) Enterovirus 71 isolated from cases of epidemic poliomyelitis-like disease in Bulgaria. *Archives in Virology,* **60**, 329–340.

Ciocca, M. (2000) Clinical course and consequences of hepatitis A infection. *Vaccine,* **18**(1), S71–S74.

Clements, G.B., Galbraith, D.N. and Taylor, K.W. (1995) Coxsackie B virus infection and onset of childhood diabetes. *The Lancet,* **346,** 221–223.

Crabtree, P.A., Gerba, K.D., Rose, C.P., J.B and Haas, C.N. (1997) Waterborne adenovirus: a risk assessment. *Water Science and Technology,* **35**(11–12), 1–6.

Crowcroft, N.S., Walsh, B., Davison, K.L. and Gungabissoon, U. (2001) Guidelines for the control of hepatitis A virus infection. *Communicable Disease and Public Health,* **4**(3), 213–227.

Cuthbert, J.A. (2001) Hepatitis A: old and new. *Clinical Microbiology Reviews,* **14**(1), 38–58.

D'Alessio D., Minor T.E., Allen C.I., Tsiatis A.A., Nelson D.B. (1981) A study of the proportions of swimmers among well controls and children with enterovirus-like illness shedding or not shedding an enterovirus. *American Journal of Epidemiology,* **113,** 533–541.

D'Angelo, L.J., Hierholzer, J.C., Keenlyside, R.A., Anderson, L.J. and Martone, W.J. (1979) Pharyngo-conjunctival fever caused by adenovirus type 4: Recovery of virus from pool water. *Journal of Infectious Diseases,* **140,** 42–47.

Debord, T. and Buisson, Y. (1998) Viral hepatitis of enteric origin. *Bulletin de la Société de Pathologie Exotique,* **91**(5 part 1–2), 428–431.

Debray, D., Cullufi, P., Devictor, D., Fabre, M. and Bernard, O. (1997) Liver failure in children with hepatitis A. *Hepatology,* **26,** 1018–1022.

Denis, F.A., Blanchouin, E., de Lignieres, A. and Flamen, P. (1974) Letter: Coxsackie A16 infection from lake water. *Journal of American Waterworks Association,* **228**(11), 1370–1371.

Dery, P., Marks, M. and Shapera, R. (1974) Clinical manifestations of coxsackievirus infections in children. *American Journal of Diseases of Children,* **128,** 464–468.

Diaz-Horta, O., Bello, M., Cabrera-Rode, E., Suarez, J., Mas, P., Garcia, I., Abalos, I., Jofre, R., Molina, G., Diaz-Diaz, O. and Dimario, U. (2001) Echovirus 4 and type 1 diabetes mellitus. *Autoimmunity,* **34**(4), 275–281.

Dorfman, M. (2004) *The growing problem of sewage pollution and how the Bush administration is putting our health and environment at risk.* National Resources Defense Council and the Environmental Integrity Project. New York. 67pp.

Edwards, K.M, Thompson, J., Paolini, J. and Wright, P.F. (1985) Adenovirus infections in young children. *Pediatrics,* **76,** 420–424.

Enriquez, C.E. and Gerba, C.P. (1995) Concentration of enteric adenovirus 40 from tap, sea and waste water. *Water Research,* **29**(11), 2554–2560.

Euscher, E., Davis, J., Holzman, I. and Nuovo, G.J. (2001) Coxsackie virus infection of the placenta associated with neurodevelopmental delays in the newborn. *Obstetrics & Gynecology,* **98**(6), 1019–1026

Foy, H.M. (1997) Adenoviruses. In: *Viral infections in humans,* 4th edn, (ed. A.S. Evans and R.A. Kaslow), pp. 119–138, New York: Plenum Press, Gaydos CA, USA.

Foy, H.M., Cooney, M.K. and Hatlen, J.B. (1968) Adenovirus type 3 epidemic associated with intermittent chlorination of a swimming pool. *Archives of Environmental Health,* **17,** 795–802.

Franklin, E.C. (1978) Arthralgias and arthritis in viral infections. *American Family Physician,* **17**(1), 161–166.

Froeschle, J.E., Feorino, P.M. and Gelfand, H.M. (1966) A continuing surveillance of enterovirus infections in healthy children in six United States cities. II. Surveillance enterovirus isolates 1960–1963 and comparison with enterovirus isolates from cases of acute central nervous system disease. *American Journal of Epidemiology,* **83**, 455.

Gammie, A.J. and Wyn-Jones, A.P. (1997) Does hepatitis A pose a significant health risk to recreational water users? *Water Science and Technology,* **35**(11–12), 171–177.

Garin, D., Fuchs, F., Crance, J.M., Rouby, Y., Chapalain, J.C., Lamarque, D., Gounot, A.M. and Aymard, M. (1994) Exposure to enteroviruses and hepatitis A virus among divers in environmental waters in France, first biological and serological survey of a controlled cohort. *Epidemiology and Infection,* **113**(3), 541–549.

Gaydos, J.C. (1999) Adenovirus vaccines. In: *Vaccines,* 3rd edn, (ed. S.A. Plotkin and W.A. Orenstein), pp. 609–628, WB Saunders: Philadelphia, USA.

Gauntt, C. and Huber, S. (2003) Coxsackievirus experimental heart diseases. *Frontiers in Bioscience,* **8**, e23–35.

Gerba, C.P., Rose, J.B. and Haas, C.N. (1996) Sensitive populations: who is at the greatest risk? *International Journal of Food Microbiology,* **30**(1-2), 113–123.

Górska, A., Urban, M., Gowiska, B. and Kowalewski, M. (1998) Is infection with group A streptococcus the only reason for rheumatic fever? – a case report of rheumatic fever coexisting with coxsackie B1 virus infection. *Przeglad Lekarski,* **55**(7–8), 418–419.

Grasland, A., Le Maitre, F., Pouchot, J., Hazera, P., Bazin, C. and Vinceneux, P. (1998) Adult-onset Still's disease after hepatitis A and B vaccination? *La Revue de Médecine Interne,* **19**(2), 134–136.

Grimwood, K., Carzino, R., Barnes, G.L. and Bishop, R.F. (1995) Patients with enteric adenovirus gastroenteritis admitted to an Australian pediatric teaching hospital from 1981 to 1992. *Journal of Clinical Microbiology,* **33**, 131–136.

Grimwood, K., Huang, Q.S., Sadleir, L,G., Nix, W.A., Kilpatrick, D.R., Oberste, M.S. and Pallansch, M.A. (2003) Acute flaccid paralysis from echovirus type 33 infection. *Journal of Clinical Microbiology,* **4**(5), 2230–2232.

Haqshenas, G., Shivaprasad, H.L., Woolcock, P.L., Read, D.H. and Meng, X.J. (2001) Genetic identification and characterization of a novel virus related to human hepatitis E virus from chickens with hepatitis-splenomegaly syndrome in the United States. *Journal of General Virology,* **82**(10), 2449–2462.

Hardy K.A, Schidlow D.V. and Zaeri, N. (1988) Obliterative bronchiolitis in children. *Chest,* **93**, 460–466.

Harley, D., Harrower, B., Lyon, M. and Dick, A. (2001) A primary school outbreak of pharyngoconjunctival fever caused by adenovirus type 3. *Communicable Diseases Intelligence,* **25**(1), 9–12.

Harrison, T.J. (1999) Hepatitis E virus – an update. *Liver,* **19**(3), 171–176.

Hawley, H.B., Morin, D.P., Geraghty, M.E., Tomkow, J. and Phillips, C.A. (1973) Coxsackievirus B epidemic at a boys' summer camp. Isolation of virus from swimming water. *Journal of American Waterworks Association,* **226**, 33–36.

Health Canada (2001) *Material data safety sheet – infectious substances.* Available on-line. http://www.hc-sc.gc.ca/pphb-dgspsp/msds-ftss/index.html#menu.

Health Canada (2002) *Material data safety sheet – infectious agents.* Available on-line: http://www.hc-sc.gc.ca/pphb-dgspsp/msds-ftss/msds3e.html.

Heinz, F., Bindas, B., Cervenka, P. and Zdebska, E. (1977) Epidemics of swimming pool conjunctivitis caused by adenovirus type 3. *Ceskoslovenska Epidemiologie, Mikrobiologie, Immunologie,* **25**(6), 321–325.

Hierholzer, J.C. (1992) Adenovirus in the immunocompromised host. *Clinics in Microbiological Reviews,* **5**, 262–274.

Hlavová, H. (1989) Coxsackie A virus infections. *Ceskoslovenska Epidemiologie, Mikrobiologie, Imunologie,* **38**(2), 74–81.

Hoeprich, P.D. (ed.) (1977) *Infectious Diseases.* 2nd edn, Harper & Row Publishers, New York, San Francisco, London.

Hogg, J. (2000) Latent adenoviral infection in the pathogenesis of emphysema. *Chest,* **117**, 282S–285S.

Hollinger, F.B. and Ticehurst, J.R. (1996) Hepatitis A virus. In: *Fields Virology,* 3rd edn, pp 735–782, Lippincott-Raven, Philadelphia, USA.

Hoofnagle, J.H., Carithers, R.L., Shapiro, C. and Ascher, N. (1995) Fulminant hepatic failure: summary of a workshop. *Hepatology,* **21**, 240–252.

Horwitz, M.S., Ilic, A., Fine, C., Balasa, B. and Sarvetnick, N. (2004) Coxsackieviral-mediated diabetes: induction requires antigen-presenting cells and is accompanied by phagocytosis of beta cells. *Clinical Immunology,* **110**(2), 134–144.

Hou, J., Said, C., Franchi, D., Franchi, D., Dockstader, P. and Chatterjee, N.K. (1994) Antibodies to glutamic acid decarboxylase and P2-C peptides in sera from coxsackie virus B4-infected mice and IDDM patients. *Diabetes,* **43**, 1260–1266.

Ho-Yen, D.O., Hardie, R., McClure, J., Cunningham, N.E. and Bell, E.J. (1989) Fatal outcome of echovirus 7 infection. *Scandanavian Journal of Infectious Diseases,* **21**, 459–461.

Hugues, B., Pietri, C., Puel, D., Crance, J.M., Cini, C. and Deloince, R. (1988) Research of enterovirus, hepatitis A virus in a bathing area over a six-month-period and their salubrity impact. *Zentralblatt Fur Bakteriologie Mikrobiologie und Hygiene,* **185**(6), 560–568.

Hunter, P.R. (1998) *Waterborne Disease. Epidemiology and Ecology.* John Wiley and Son Ltd, Chichester, UK.

Hyöty, H. and Taylor, K.W. (2002) The role of viruses in human diabetes. *Diabetologia,* **45**(10), 1353–1361.

Inge, T., Philippe, L., Van Der Donck, I., Beuselinck, K., Lindberg, A.M. and Van Ranst, M. (2003) Molecular typing and epidemiology of enteroviruses identified from an outbreak of aseptic meningitis in Belgium during the summer of 2000. *Journal of Medical Virology,* **70**(3), 420–429.

Jaeckel, E., Manns, M. and Von Herrath, M. (2002) Viruses and diabetes. *Annals of the New York Academy of Sciences,* **958**, 7.

Jaiswal, S.P.B., Jain, A.K., Naik, G., Soni, N. and Chitnis, D.S. (2001) Viral hepatitis during pregnancy. *International Journal of Gynecology & Obstretrics,* **72**(2), 103–108.

Karetnyi, Y.V., Gilchrist, M.J.R. and Naides, S.J. (1999) Hepatitis E virus infection prevalence among selected populations in Iowa. *Journal of Clinical Virology,* **14**(1), 51–55.

Kazi, N.J., Cepeda, E.E. and Budev, H. (1988) Fatal echovirus type 7 in a premature infant. *American Journal of Perinatology,* **5**(3), 236–238.

Kee, F., McElroy, G., Stewart, D., Coyle, P and Watson, J. (1994) A community outbreak of echovirus infection associated with an outdoor swimming pool. *Journal of Public Health Medicine*, **16**, 145–148.

Keswick B.H., Gerba, C.P. and Goyal, S.M. (1981) Occurrence of enteroviruses in community swimming pools. *American Journal of Public Health*, **71**(9), 1026–1030.

Khuroo, M.S., Teli, M.R., Skidmore, S.S., Sofi, M.A. and Khuroo, M.I. (1981) Incidence and severity of viral hepatitis in pregnancy. *American Journal of Medicine, 70*, 252–255.

King, A.M.Q., Brown, F., Christian, P., Hovi, T., Hyypiä, T., Knowles, N.J., Lemon, S.M., Minor, P.D., Palmenberg, A.C., Skern, T. and Stanway, G. (2000) *Picornaviradae*. In: *Virus Taxonomy, Seventh Report of the International Committee for the Taxonomy of Viruses* (ed. M.H.V. Van Regenmortel, C.M. Fauquet, D.H.L. Bishop, C.H. Calisher, E.B. Carsten, M.K. Estwes, S.M. Lemon, J. Maniloff, M.A. Mayo, D.J. McGeoch, C.R. Pringle, and R.B. Wickner), pp.657–673, Academic Press, New York, San Diego, USA.

Kitamura, N. (2001) Genome analysis of adenovirus type 7 and adenovirus type 11. *Japanese Journal of Ophthalmology, 45*(1), 22–30.

Kono, R., Miyamura, K., Tajiri, E., Sasgawa, A. and Phuapradit, P. (1977) Virological and serological studies of neurological complications of acute hemorrhagic conjunctivitis in Thailand. *Journal of Infectious Diseases*, **135**, 706–713.

Koontz, C.H. and Ray, C.G. (1971) The role of coxsackievirus B infections in sporadic myopericarditis. *American Heart Journal*, **82**(6), 750–758.

Kopecka, H., Dubrou, S., Prevot, J. Marechal, J. and Lopez-Pila, J.M. (1993) Detection of naturally occurring enteroviruses in water by reverse transcription, polymerase chain reaction, and hybridization. *Applied Environmental Microbiology*, **59**, 1213–1219.

Ledner, W.M., Lemon, S.M., Kirkpatrick, J.W., Redfield, R.R., Fields, M.L. and Kelley, P.W. (1985). Frequency of illness associated with epidemic hepatitis A virus infections in adults. *American Journal of Epidemiology, 122*, 226–233.

Lemon, S.M. (1995) Hepatitis E virus. In: Mandell, G.L., Bennett, J.E. and Dolin, R. (eds). *Principles and Practice of Infectious Diseases*, 4th edn. New York, Churchill Livingstone. 1663–1666.

Leslie, R.D. and Elliott, R.B. Early environmental events as a cause of IDDM. Evidence and implications. *Diabetes, 43*(7), 843-850.

Lucht, F., Alexandre, C., Fayard, C., Gaudin, O.G. and Mathevet, N. (1984) Athritis associated with coxsackie B virus infections. *Revue du Rhumatisme et des Maladies Osteo-Articulaires*, **51**(3), 153–155.

Macek V., Sorli J., Kopriva S. and Marin J. (1994) Persistent adenoviral infection and chronic airway obstruction in children. *American Journal of Respiratory and Critical Care Medicine, 150*, 7.

Madhaven, H.N. and Sharma, K.B. (1969) Enterovirus from cases of encephalitis in Pondicherry. *Indian Journal of Medical Research*, **57**, 1607–1610.

Madhi, S. A., Schoub, B. Simmank, K. Blackburn, N. Klugman, K. P. (2000) Increased burden of respiratory viral associated severe lower respiratory tract infections in children infected with human immunodeficiency virus type-1. *The Journal of Pediatrics, 137*(1), 78–84.

Mahoney, F.J., Farley, T.A., Kelso, K.Y., Wilson, S.A., Horan, J.M. and McFarland, L.M. (1992) An outbreak of hepatitis A associated with swimming in a public pool. *Journal of Infectious Diseases*, **165**, 613–618.

Mandell, G.L. (2000) *Principles and Practice of Infectious Diseases*. Churchill Livingstone.

Martone, W.J., Hierholzer, J.C., Keenlyside, R.A., Fraser, DW., D'Angelo, L.J. and Winkler, W.G. (1980) An outbreak of adenovirus type 3 disease at a private recreation center swimming pool. *American Journal of Epidemiology*, **111**, 229–237.

Marzouk, Y., Goyal, S.M. and Gerba, C.P. (1980) Relationship of viruses and indicator bacteria in water and wastewater of Israel. *Water Research*, **14**(11), 1585–1590.

McAbee, G.N. and Kadakia, S. (2001) A child with Coxsackie A3 encephalitis. *Pediatric Neurology*, **25**(1), 84.

Mena, I., Fischer, C., Gebhard, J.R., Perry, C.M., Harkins, S. and Whitton, J.L. (2000) Coxsackievirus infection of the pancreas: evaluation of receptor expression, pathogenesis, and immunopathology. *Virology*, **271**, 276–288.

Mena, K.D., Gerba, C.P., Haas, C.N. and Rose, J.B. (2003) Risk assessment of waterborne coxsackievirus. *Journal of the American Water Works Association*, **95**(7), 122–131.

Mena, I., Perry, C.M., Harkins, S., Rodriguez, F., Gebhard, J. and Whitton, J.L. (1999) The role of B lymphocytes in coxsackievirus B3 infection. *American Journal of Pathology*, **155**, 1205–1215.

Meng, X.J., Purcell, R.H., Halbur, P.G., Lehman, J.R., Webb, D.M. and Tsareva, T.S. (1997) A novel virus in swine is closely related to the human hepatitis E virus. *Proceedings of the National Academy of Sciences of the United States of America*, **94**, 9860–9865.

Metcalf, T.G., Melnick, J.L. and Estes, M.K. (1995) Environmental virology: from detection of virus in sewage and water by isolation to identification by molecular biology – a trip of over 50 years. *Annual Review of Microbiology*, **49**, 461–487.

Mickan, L.D. and Kok, T.W. (1994) Recognition of adenovirus types in faecal samples by southern hybridization in South Australia. *Epidemiology and Infection*, **112**(3), 603–613.

Minor, P. (1998) *Picornaviruses*. In: *Topley and Wilson's Microbiology and Microbial Infections*. Hodder Arnold, London, UK.

Mirghani, O.A., Saeed, O.K. and Basama, F.M. (1992) Viral hepatitis in pregnancy. *East African Medical Journal*, **69**, 445–449.

Mishra, A., Saigal, A., Gupta, R. and Sarin, S.K. (1999) Acute pancreatitis associated with viral hepatitis: a report of six cases with review of literature. *The American Journal of Gastroenterology*, **94**(8), 2292–2295.

Murray, C.J.L. and Lopez, A.D. (1996) Evidence based health policy: lessons from the global burden of disease study. *Science*, **274**, 740–743.

Murtagh, P., Cerqueiro, C., Halac, A., Avila, M. and Kajon, A. (1993) Adenovirus type 7h respiratory infections. A report of 29 cases of acute lower respiratory disease. *Acta Paediatrica*, **82**, 557–561.

Murtagh, P. and Kajon, A. (1997) Chronic pulmonary sequelae of adenovirus infection. *Pediatric Pulmonology. Supplement*, **16**, 150–151.

Muscillo, M., La Rosa, G., Aulicino, F.A., Orsini, P., Bellucci, C. and Micarelli, R. (1995) Comparison of cDNA probe hybridizations and RT-PCR detection methods for the identification and differentiation of enteroviruses isolated from sea water samples. *Water Research,* **29**(5), 1309–1316.

Ohori, N.P., Michaels, M.G., Jaffe, R., Williams, P. and Yousem, S.A. (1995) Adenovirus pneumonia in lung transplant recipients. *Human Pathology,* **26**, 1073–1079.

Otonkoski, T., Roivainen, M., Vaarala, O., Dinesen, B., Leipälä, J.A., Hovi, T. and Knip, M. (2000) Neonatal Type I diabetes associated with maternal echovirus 6 infection: a case report. *Diabetologia,* **43**(10), 1235–1238.

Palambo, E.A. and Bishop, R.F. (1996) Annual incidence, serotype distribution, and genetic diversity of human astrovirus isolates from hospitalized children in Melbourne, Australia. *Journal of Clinical Microbiology,* **34**, 1750–1753.

Panà, A., Divizia, M., De Filippis, P. and Di Napoli, A. (1987) Isolation of hepatitis A virus from polluted river water on FRP/3 cells. *Lancet,* **330**(8571), 1328.

Papapetropoulou, M. and Vantarakis, A.C. (1998) Detection of adenovirus outbreak at a municipal swimming pool by nested PCR amplification. *The Journal of Infection,* **36**(1), 101–103.

Payment, P. (1991) Antibody levels to selected enteric viruses in a normal randomly selected Canadian population. *Immunology and Infectious Diseases,* **1**, 317–322.

Percival, S.L., Chalmer, R.M., Embrey, M., Hunter, P.R., Sellwood, J. and Wyn-Jones, P. (2004) *Microbiology of waterborne diseases.* Elsevier Academic Press, Great Britain. 480pp.

Pongpanich, B., Boonpucknavig, S., Wasi, C., Tanphaichitr, P. and Boonpucknavig, V. (1983) Immunopathology of acute rheumatic fever and rheumatic heart disease. The demonstration of Coxsackie group B viral antigen in the myocardium. *Clinical Rheumatology,* **2**(3), 217–222.

Powledge, T.M. (2004) Is obesity an infectious disease? *The Lancet Infectious Diseases,* **4**(10), 599.

Purcell, R.H. (1995) Hepatitis viruses: changing patterns of human disease. In: Roizman, B (ed.). *Infectious diseases in an age of change.* Washington DC, National Academy Press, 59–75.

Ramia, A. (1985) Transmission of viral infections by the water route: Implications for developing countries. *Review of Infectious Diseases,* **7**(2), 180–188.

Ramsingh, A.I., Chapman, N.M. and Tracy, S. (1997) Coxsackievirus and diabetes. *Bioessays,* **19**, 793–800.

Reichier, M.R., Valway, S.E. and Onorato I.M. (2000) Acute hepatitis E infection acquired in California. *Clinical Infectious Diseases,* **30**, 618–619.

Rosenberg, M.L., Koplan, J.P. and Pollard, R.A. (1980) The risk of acquiring hepatitis from sewage-contaminated water. *American Journal of Epidemiology,* **112**(1), 17–22.

Rose, J.B., Mullinax, R.L., Singh, S.N., Yates, M.V. and Gerba, C.P. (1987) Occurrence of rotaviruses and enteroviruses in recreational waters of Oak Creek, Arizona. *Water Research,* **21**(11), 1375–1381.

Ruuskanen, O., Meurman, O. and Sarkkinen, H. (1985) Adenoviral diseases in children. A study of 105 hospital cases. *Pediatrics,* **76**, 79–83.

Schiff, E.R. (1992) Atypical clinical manifestations of hepatitis A. *Vaccine,* **10**(1), S18–S20.

Schvoerer, E., Bonnet, F., Dubois, V., Cazaux, G., Serceau, R., Fleury, H. and Lafon, M.E. (2000) PCR detection of human enteric viruses in bathing areas, waste waters and human stools in south-western France. *Research in Microbiology,* **151,** 693–701.

See Lum, L.C., Chua, K.B., McMinn, P.C., Goh, A.Y.T., Muridan, R., Sarji, S.A., Hooi, P.S., Chua, B.H. and Lam, S.K. (2002) Echovirus 7 associated encephalomyelitis, *Journal of Clinical Virology,* **23**(3), 153–160.

Sharp I.R. and Wadell G. (1995) Adenoviruses. In: Zukerman AJ, Banatvalla J, Pattison JR, (eds). *Principles and Practice of Clinical Virology,* 3rd. edn. New York: Wiley, 287–308.

Shuval, H.I. (1988) The transmission of virus disease by the marine environment. *Schriftenreihe Des Vereins Fur Wasser-, Boden-Und Lufthygiene,* **78,** 7–23.

Simila, S., Linna, O., Lanning, P., Heikkinen, E. and Ala-Houhala, M. (1981) Chronic lung damage caused by adenovirus type 7. A ten-year follow-up study. *Chest,* **80,** 127–131.

Simsir, A., Greenebaum, E., Nuovo, G. and Schulman, L.L. (1998) Late fatal adenovirus pneumonitis in a lung transplant recipient. *Transplantation,* **65,** 592–594.

Sly, P.D., Soto-Quiros, M.E., Landau, L.I., Hudson, I. and Newton-John, H. (1984) Factors predisposing to abnormal pulmonary function after adenovirus type 7 pneumonia. *Archives of Disease in Childhood,* **59,** 935–939.

Sobsey, M. D., Shields, P. A., Hauchman, F. S., Davis, A. L., Rullman, V. A. and Bosch, A. (1988). Survival and persistence of hepatitis A virus in environmental samples. In: A. J. Zuckerman (ed) *Viral hepatitis and liver diseases,* pp. 121–124. New York: Alan R. Liss.

Sun, C.J. and Duara, S. (1985) Fatal adenovirus pneumonia in two newborn infants, one caused by adenovirus type 30. *Pediatatric Pathology,* **4,** 247–255.

Suresh, L., Chandrasekar, S., Rao, R.S., Ravi, V. and Badrinath, S. (1989) Coxsackie virus and rheumatic fever. A correlative study. *The Journal of the Association of Physicians of India,* **37**(9), 582–585.

Tallis, G. and Gregory, J. (1997) An outbreak of hepatitis A associated with a spa pool. *Communicable Disease Intelligence,* **21**(23), 353–354.

Tan, W.C., Xiang, X., Qiu, D., Ng, T.P., Lam, S.F. and Hegele, R.G. (2003) Epidemiology of respiratory viruses in patients hospitalised with near-fatal asthma, acute exacerbations of asthma, or chronic obstructive pulmonary disease. *The American Journal of Medicine,* **115**(4), 272–277.

Taylor, M.B., Becker, P.J., Janse van Rensburg, E., Harris, B., Bailey, I.W. and Grabow, W.O.K. (1995) A serosurvey of water-borne pathogens amongst canoeists in South Africa. *Epidemiology and Infection,* **115,** 299–307.

Taylor, M.B., Cox, N., Vrey, M.A. and Grabow, W.O.K. (2001) The occurrence of hepatitis A and astrovirus in selected river and dam waters in South Africa. *Water Research,* **35**(11), 2653–2660.

Tei, S., Kitajima, N., Takahashi, K. and Mishiro, S. (2003) Zoonotic transmission of hepatitis E virus from deer to human beings. *The Lancet,* **362**(9381), 371–373.

Thompson, S.S., Jackson, J.L., Suva-Castillo, M., Yanko, W.A., El Jack, Z., Kuo, J.C.C., Williams, F.P. and Schnurr, D.P. (2003) Detection of infectious human adenoviruses in tertiary-treated and ultraviolet-disinfected wastewater. *Water*

Environment Research: a Research Publication of the Water Environment Federation, **75**(2), 163–170.

Thurston-Enriquez, J.A., Haas, C.N., Jacangelo, J., Riley, K. and Gerba, C.P. (2003) Inactivation of feline calicivirus and adenovirus type 40 by UV radiation. *Applied and Environmental Microbiology,* **69**(1), 577–582.

Tsao, K.C., Chang, P.Y., Ning, H.C., Sun, C.F., Lin. T.Y., Chang, L.Y., Huang, Y.C. and Shih, S.R. (2002) Use of molecular assay in diagnosis of hand, foot and mouth disease caused by enterovirus 71 or coxsackievirus A 16. *Journal of Virological Methods,* **102**(1–2), 9–14.

Turner, M., Istre, G.R., Beauchamp, H., Baum, M. and Arnold, S. (1987) Community outbreak of adenovirus type 7a infections associated with a swimming pool. *Southern Medical Journal,* **80**, 712–715.

Uysal, G., Ozkaya, E. and Guvan, A. (2000) Echovirus 30 outbreak of aseptic meningitis in Turkey. *Pediatric Disease Journal,* **19**, 490.

Videla, C., Carballal, G., Misirlian, A. and Aguila, M. (1998) Acute lower respiratory infections due to respiratory syncytial virus and adenovirus among hospitalised children from Argentina. *Clinical Diagnostic Virology,* **10**, 17–23.

Viquesnel, G., Vabret, A., Leroy, G., Bricard, H. and Quesnel, J. (1997) Severe adenovirus type 7 pneumonia in a immunocompetent adult. *Annales Françaises d'Anesthésie et de Réanimation,* **16**(1), 50–52.

Ward, S. (2001) Complement modulates induction of autoimmune myocarditis. *Trends in Immunology,* **22**(10), 544.

WHO (1979) *Report of WHO Scientific Group of human viruses in water, wastewater and soil. Technical Report Series,* no. 639. World Health Organization, Geneva, Switzerland.

WHO (2000) Hepatitis A. *WHO Department of Communicable Disease Surveillance and Response, Geneva.* WHO/CDS/CSR/EDC/2000.7.

WHO (2002) State of the art of new vaccines: research and development. Diarrhoeal diseases. Available on-line: http://www.who.int/vaccine_research/documents/new_vaccines/en/index1.html. Accessed 14th July 2005.

WHO (2003) http://www.who.int/vaccines/en/hepatitisa.shtml.

WHO (2004) *Guidelines for drinking-water quality.* Volume 1: Recommendations. 3rd edn, World Health Organization, Geneva.

Wilhelmi, I., Roman, E. and Sanchez-Fauquier, A. (2003) Viruses causing gastroenteritis. *Clinical Microbiology and Infection: The Official Publication of the European Society of Clinical Microbiology and Infectious Diseases,* **9**(4), 247–262.

Wolfgram, L.J., Beisel, K.W. and Rose, N.R. (1985) Heart-specific autoantibodies following murine coxsackievirus B3 myocarditis. *Journal of Experimental Medicine,* **161**, 1112–1121.

Worm, H.C., Wim H. van der Poel, M. and Brandstätter, G. (2002) Hepatitis E: an overview. *Microbes and Infection,* **4**(6), 657–666.

Wreghitt, T.G., Sutehall, G.M., King, A. and Gandy, G.M. (1989) Fatal echovirus 7 infection during an outbreak in a special care baby unit. *Journal of Infection,* **19**, 229–236.

Yamadera, S., Yamshita, K., Akatsuka, M., Kato, N and Inouye, S. (1998) Trend of adenovirus type 7 infection, an emerging disease in Japan: a report of the National

Epidemiological Surveillance of Infectious Agents in Japan. *Japanese Journal of Medical Science and Biology,* **51**, 43–51.

Yin-Murphy, M. and Lim, K.H. (1972) Picornavirus epidemic conjunctivitis in Singapore. *The Lancet*, **300**(7782), 857–858.

Zaher, S.R., Kassem, A.S. and Hughes, J.J. (1993) Coxsackie virus infections in rheumatic fever. *Indian Journal of Pediatrics*, **60**(2), 289–298.

Zahradnik, J.M., Spencer, M.J. and Porter, D.D. (1980) Adenovirus infection in the immunocompromised patient. *American Journal of Medicine,* **68**, 725–732.

Zarraga, A.L., Kerns, F.T., Kitchen L.W. (1992) Adenovirus pneumonia with severe sequelae in an immunocompetent adult. *Clinical Infectious Diseases,* **15**, 712–713.

Zhi-Yi, X., Zi-Hua, L., Jian-Xiang, W., Zai-Ping, X. and De-Xiang D. (1992) Ecology and prevention of a shellfish-associated hepatitis A epidemic in Shanghai, China. *Vaccine,* **10**(1), S67–S68.

Zuckerman, J.N. (2003) Hepatitis E and the traveller. *Travel Medicine and Infectious Disease,* **1**(2), 73–76.

Index